SUCCESS WITH HEART FAILURE

SUCCESS WITH HEART FAILURE

Help and Hope for Those with Congestive Heart Failure

THIRD EDITION

Marc A. Silver, M.D.

Foreword by Lynne Warner Stevenson, M.D.

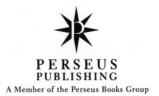

PERSEUS
PUBLISHING
A Member of the Perseus Books Group

Cataloging-in-Publication Data is available from the Library of Congress.

ISBN 0-7382-0600-8

Perseus Publishing is a Member of the Perseus Books Group.

Find us on the World Wide Web at http://www.perseuspublishing.com

Perseus Publishing books are available at special discounts for bulk purchases in the U.S. by corporations, institutions, and other organizations. For more information, please contact the Special Markets Department at the Perseus Books Group, 11 Cambridge Center, Cambridge, MA 02142, or call (800) 255-1514 or (617) 252-5298, or e-mail j.mccrary@perseusbooks.com.

Text design by Trish Wilkinson
Set in 10.5-point AGaramond by the Perseus Books Group

First printing, September 2002

1 2 3 4 5 6 7 8 9 10—06 05 04 03 02

To my patients—who have helped me learn how to help them make a Success out of Heart Failure.

Contents

Foreword

Here is a common condition with an unfortunate name. Most patients who carry that diagnosis have hearts that function well enough most of the time to sustain daily lives that are enjoyable and meaningful, as outlined in this book. These hearts are handicapped, but not defeated. In the developed countries, and particularly in the United States, there is an obsession with the ideal, both in body and in mind, that denies the universality of imperfection. Most adults have chronic health conditions that limit their lives some of the time, and heart failure is one of these.

Success with Heart Failure helps to return confidence and vitality to patients and those who care about them but may have become discouraged by their actual experiences and their greater fears about heart failure. This book also demonstrates the profound connection that can develop between those providing and those receiving medical care, when they work to exchange and enhance their understanding.

The fundamental lessons learned from heart failure are those taught by any chronic condition associated with adversity and death, of which the most common is life itself. One of the first lessons is that afflictions are not a punishment for something done or not done. We have only to walk through a pediatric cancer ward to realize the egocentric error of assuming that we have earned our fortunes.

A later challenge is how to give up the search for safety. A thorough understanding of the heart failure condition includes recognition that death, when it finally comes, may occur suddenly, at any time, without warning. Patients and their companions initially yearn for the time when life seemed secure. It takes more time to recognize the fundamental uncertainty that life was never and will never be secure for anyone. Indeed, experience with heart failure may give us a head start toward coming to terms with the transience that infuses a richness into each day, which will never come again.

Everyone who hears or delivers the diagnosis of heart failure is reminded of the limits and lack of limits of our own power. No amount of familiarity with the suits will allow us to pick the cards that we are dealt. We are, however, in control of how we arrange and play our hand. Just as the body can aggravate or ease the burdens of heart failure by physiologic responses to the changing circulation, so our own focus and attitudes influence the lives we live with our conditions. This book proves again that knowledge is power, and encourages us to take charge of all those aspects of heart failure that can be controlled.

It is vital to embrace rather than to abandon the intrinsic rhythms, marked by celebrations and vacations as well as ordinary time. Reach out and plan for those that are the most important, and the apparent logistic difficulties can usually be surmounted. For those pleasures that must routinely be denied, never say never, but promise yourself the rare indulgence. Avoid attributing all of the struggles to heart failure, and avoid seeking explanations for all of the syncopation; we must remember that there have always been days that are better or worse than others.

Perhaps most of all, this book addresses those thoughts that come in the middle of the night to those who fight breathlessness, to those who hear them fighting, and to those who do not. This book reminds and reassures all of us that we are not alone.

LYNNE WARNER STEVENSON, M.D.
Clinical Director, Cardimyopathy and Heart Failure
Cardiomyopathy and Transplant Center
Brigham and Women's Hospital
Associate Professor of Medicine, Harvard Medical School

Preface to the New Edition

And so my threat of writing yet another edition of *Success with Heart Failure* has been fulfilled. Similar motivations were the driving forces for this *final* edition. There have been new advances in the diagnosis and treatment of heart failure that I thought were sufficient to include in an updated version. Also, though the degree of public awareness has grown it is nowhere near the level needed to change heart failure from being a national health care problem into a forgotten disease that medical students will only read about in books.

However, if public awareness alone was my goal, I would have only spent even more of my time on the Heart Failure Awareness activities of the Heart Failure Society of America. This organization, which I helped found, has become a vital force for heart failure activities throughout North America (http://www.hfsa.org). One of the key areas the society has undertaken in recent years is a variety of attempts to increase the public and professional awareness of heart failure and the advances being made each day. However, even acknowledging that progress in public awareness takes time. I was convinced that no single paths or series of approaches can adequately address the immediate need for useful public information about heart failure.

In the end, however, the final motivation to write this updated edition came not from the need to discuss the advances nor from the ever-present need for public awareness. The true story is this; I have pictures of several of my patients that I have taken over the years. About six months ago I put these pictures in a file on my computer. I have used this file of pictures as my screen saver. So when I get up in the morning or go to work on the computer in the wee hours of night, the first things I see are the pictures of these patients. I see the face of the young mother who had peripartum cardiomyopathy (who was told never to have any children) who is now seen posing with her two young boys, or the couple now married fifty-five years—the husband came to me eight years ago near death—who now live and enjoy each day together, or the man who, thanks to participation in our trials for advanced heart failure, is seen kissing his wife. It is these reminders that are the true motivation for this edition. They tell me they couldn't have done it without me and in fact I couldn't have done it without them. Their strength and courage goes beyond heroics and simply speaks to the fact that despite what you have heard, no matter how you feel, there can be *success with heart failure!*

And so I wish you well on your journey. If this book has helped you (as the hundreds and hundreds of letters I have received indicate) then share what you have learned with anyone who might benefit—your friends, neighbors, doctors, and nurses. It is only when we share the common belief that something can be done for almost everyone with heart failure that we will be on the real road to *success!*

Marc A. Silver, M.D.
April 2002

How to Read This Book

This book is organized into sections: discussing what heart failure is, how one gets it, how it's diagnosed, how it's treated, and so forth. I have tried to make the flow as natural and logical as possible. I have also tried to make this book readable for everyone who picks it up. Therefore, I have made an attempt to explain some of the complex concepts regarding heart failure and cardiac physiology and pathology in terms that everyone will understand. On the other hand, I've tried not to make it so simple that other health care professionals will dismiss it and not find anything useful in it.

The reader may find some redundancy, since several of the key concepts in treating heart failure recur throughout the book. Finally, I have included several appendixes at the end of the book that provide more detail, including photographs of hearts, and list references the reader will find useful.

I think you will find it useful before plunging into the main chapters to read the introduction, and to then take a moment and look through Appendix I, which is a glossary of heart failure terms. This should help familiarize you with some of the terms that are used and may provide a basis for understanding as you begin to read the text. As you read through the text, you may want to stop and consult the appendixes to look up a term, to check a drug, or to look at some of the photographs I have included.

I hope you will use this book as I have intended it—as a resource that you can return to time and again to enhance your understanding of heart failure.

Acknowledgments

The number of people to thank has grown to be innumerable. Nevertheless, I again want to make an attempt to mention those who have helped me and are, in fact, the stuff of which this book is made. As I said in the first edition, however, if after reading this book you do not find it useful or helpful for yourself or for a friend or relative, consider the book, in its entirety, my doing. On the other hand, if you gain some knowledge, some insight, or some hope for yourself or a loved one, recognize that the people mentioned in the following paragraphs are some of those who made it happen.

My deepest gratitude goes to my beloved parents, my late father, Sam, and my dear mother, Ida, who brought me into this world to do something good—I hope I have, at least in part, fulfilled their dreams—and to my "younger" sister, Betty Ann, and her family, who have been a support always. I appreciate all the help Betty Ann gave me along the way; she will never know why I think she is the strong one.

My patients have been a constant source of knowledge and support. In sharing their hearts and emotions with me, they have given me a great gift. Some have asked me to teach them about heart failure and made me become a better doctor. Others have taught me lessons about heart failure that no medical school or textbooks could. Others have taught me how precious life and hope are—lessons I pray I will not forget.

On a daily basis, I am grateful for the work I do, and even more grateful that I have had dedicated nursing professionals working with me over the years with the expertise and vision to better the lives of those who have heart failure.

Special appreciation goes to all the nurses of the Heart Failure Institute at Advocate Christ Medical Center; these include Carol Pisano, Helen Lonergan-Thomas, Sharon Brennan, Kate Karns, Kathie Kamba, Melissa Gabriel, Colleen Gallagher, Eileen Golden, Cindy Knepper, Cathy McAvoy, Sue Novosel, and Linda Saveas.

Also, very special appreciation for Char Nutter, my administrative assistant who is a daily positive force in my life. Those who know me know that Char is the one who gets me through each day. I value her assistance, advice, and friendship. I also acknowledge the members of my research office, Kay Murphy, Maggie Sokolowski, Diane Braun, and Kelly Bretz, all of whom help bring new advances to our patients earlier.

Finally, the person who truly is the *success* in *Success with Heart Failure* is Pam Cianci, R.N., M.S.N. Pam is the institute's advanced practice nurse but is truly at the heart of all we do. Her enormous energy and willingness to get things done for our patients is a wonderment to me every day. So for every patient, every family member, and every referring doctor and for anyone who has had the pleasure to know Pam, I say thank you.

Thanks also to Jeannine Pfau, R.D., who helped me with sections in this book on dietary restrictions and sodium content of foods.

I also thank my mentors, including Drs. William C. Roberts, Joseph Messer, and Karl T. Weber, who showed me in words and deeds what hard work is all about. And to all my former and present colleagues at the National Heart, Lung, and Blood Institute, Rush Presbyterian St. Luke's Medical Center, the University of Chicago, the University of Illinois, Michael Reese Hospital, and Loyola University, I extend my gratitude. Also to Drs. Hugo Cuadros, Pat Pappas, Mark Slaughter, Tony Tatooles, Robert Stein, and Ms. Carol Schneider, whose vision helped me develop the Heart Failure Institute at Advocate Christ Hospital and Medical Center, I give thanks.

For Louis Le Jacq and Dr. Jay Cohn, who invited me to sit around a table with them and a handful of folks to bring forward the Heart Failure Society of America—this is a force of good in heart failure today. To all the "founding fathers" as well as to those who will follow in our steps I ask for health and energy to continue to do good work. Special thanks to Cheryl Yana, executive director of the society and strong supporter. And to Dr. John Strobeck who serves as my coeditor-in-chief of our journal, *Congestive Heart Failure*. This journal, which is the most widely circulated journal in the world focusing on heart failure, takes time and effort but again is doing good things and so John and I simply do the work that needs to be done.

I want to thank Dr. Fred Weinstein, who single-handedly did so much to help me become a physician—I don't know if I have ever thanked him enough. Dr. Robert Kark took a young intern aside for breakfast one morning and put a career on course; he, too, has probably not been thanked adequately. Also thanks to Dr. Hadi Dizadji who introduced me to the world of cardiology. I am certainly grateful to and appreciate the trust of the many physicians, both locally and from around the country, who refer patients to me for evaluation.

The first edition of this book had many passages. It sat in my head for about four years. The next passage came when my dear friends, Allan and Gail

Muehrcke, got tired of hearing about "the book" and banished me for two days to their summer cottage, where the initial chapters took form. I thank Julie R. Dunne, who helped guide this book to the next passage, putting it on the proper path toward publication. I thank the folks of Perseus, especially Marnie Cochran, my editor, and Rebecca Marks, who have continued to guide this book. I thank those friends and colleagues who critically read parts or all of the book.

Finally, for my wife, Laureen, and my children—Zachary, Adam, Nora, Ryan, Jacob, and Meredith—I am eternally grateful. They know that helping patients is a sacred duty for me and have yielded their time with me when I know it was difficult.

And to all, spoken or unspoken, in both body and spirit, who do their best to help with this disease of our nation, I give thanks. To everyone who has touched my path, I give thanks.

Introduction

The first edition of this book was written to provide an educational tool for my patients with heart failure. I tried to cram into it all the basics and put into language that was simple and understandable the core knowledge of heart failure—things that by reading alone would make them feel better, be more educated about their disease, and at the same time derive more benefit from their relationship with their doctors and nurses.

This edition is the same—and more! I have tried to not "mess" with a good thing (and that is what the thousands of letters from readers told me!). But, since the last edition, changes have come about in our understanding of heart failure, in my approaches, in medical care in general, and in how we all get and process information. This edition tries to bring *Success with Heart Failure* into the next millennium.

This book remains the primer and working text for patients and families who have or who are at risk for heart failure. It starts with the basics of describing what the terrible term is, what it means, and how it impacts lifestyles. But I have learned that it is more than that for so many. It is often the questions answered that never get asked to people's own doctors. It is the time to explain the "hows" and "whys" of heart failure symptoms in terms that make the light go on and make people say "Oh yeah, now I understand why I need to limit my salt intake!" It is the extra fifteen or twenty minutes the busy doctors or nurses don't have in these days of health care change, where treating heart failure patients has become almost punitive economically.

I hope it is, as well, the lessons and conversations that family members want to hear and get involved in as they become part of the support system for someone with heart failure.

And as we live in an age of technology explosion, then, even more than the first edition, this book serves as the guide to get more and better heart failure information in the future, long after the lessons of this edition are outdated.

As I said in the introduction to the first edition, I want you to realize that no two individuals are exactly alike, and bear in mind that only so much of the diagnosis and treatment of heart failure can be put down on a written page. Therefore, always recall my best advice, which is to corroborate and consult with your own team of doctors and nurses—those you trust and feel are interested in you—to help you decide upon the right approaches for your heart failure.

Medicine is an imperfect science and therefore neither author nor publishers can assume responsibilities for advice, omissions, or errors.

In the first edition I welcomed your feedback and provided a post office box. I cannot tell you how delighted I was to get your letters and read them all. I was not prepared for the volume and therefore could not answer many directly. Often, reams of medical records would come, and that made me feel uncomfortable. I still welcome your comments for future projects, but please understand my inability to respond.

Therefore, my thanks again to all who helped on this path, and I wish you Godspeed as you start on the path to *Success with Heart Failure*. The power is yours!

1

Don't Be Angry

As in the first edition of *Success with Heart Failure*, I have placed this chapter first. After many years of seeing patients who come to me for diagnosis and treatment of advanced symptoms of heart disease, they and I remain mystified about how this happened to them. On occasion, it is a sudden, unpredictable event. Mostly, however, heart disease is the natural, predictable path of events happening right under our noses.

I often use the analogy of how "symptomatic heart failure" occurs as the "straw that breaks the camel's back." That is, the heart, like all our organs, has so much reserve power that we can use up a lot of the reserve without noticing any symptoms; then, seemingly out of the blue, we use up that last little bit of the heart's reserve and symptoms develop. With this event, patients, families, and even doctors are surprised at how a person who felt great and was able to mow the lawn or carry groceries can be rather suddenly transformed into someone who cannot even walk up the stairs without gasping for air or having to rest.

It is this "sudden" transformation that causes a great deal of uncertainty, fear, depression, and even anger. (See Chapter 4 for a detailed discussion on depression.) That is why I begin this book with a few words about this anger.

Many years ago, when I began writing this book, this was the first chapter I wrote. I discarded it early on but later decided to include it. I feel I must say a few words about anger and emotions before I delve into other topics. Heart failure, in reality, is commonly a chronic disease process, meaning that although there is often not a complete cure, there are ways to improve and stabilize the condition and certainly better ways to understand and live with it. However, when most patients initially hear the words *heart failure*, which is indeed an unfortunate term, they equate the term with fatality, and an array of emotions emerge—or, more often, *don't* emerge—and eventually impact relationships the patient has with physicians, nurses, and family members.

We know from the important work done by Dr. Elisabeth Kübler-Ross *(On Death and Dying)* and others that when patients are told they have a terminal illness—a form of cancer, for example—they pass through several emotional stages until they reach a level of acceptance. Even when patients are told they have systemic hypertension or high blood pressure (which can be very well controlled and treated but usually requires lifelong dietary and medical therapy), a similar reaction occurs. Therefore, it is not unexpected for anger to ensue when patients learn they have heart failure. Part of the problem is a lack of understanding of what heart failure is and what can be done for it (hence, this book). However, even an insightful understanding of heart failure leads to the notion that life somehow will be different, will include more medical care, and will inevitably be shortened. Who wouldn't be angry or upset? My advice, then, really, is *do* be angry—but only for a period sufficient to work through those emotions and get more information and help. Then, don't be angry!

In general, anger is not a useful emotion unless it motivates an individual to do more to improve the situation. Once a person acts on this motivation, the knowledge and acceptance that result should eventually melt away the anger. If, instead, the anger remains, the use of any knowledge or understanding will be inhibited by this powerful emotion.

In caring for patients waiting for a heart transplant, I have observed that in those who wait prolonged periods of time for a donor to become available (and the wait nowadays often is months to years, and much of the time is spent in a hospital on support medicines and devices), the predominant emotion is anger—anger over the wait, the chronicity of their illness, and their fate in having heart disease. Moreover, they remain angry when their long-awaited goal comes to fruition, and the anger persists into the posttransplant period, preventing them from fully appreciating the gift they have received. These patients alienate family and friends and lose support systems they desperately need.

I have no magic formula for patients to learn how to work through the initial anger and let it melt away into a better understanding. In some cases, anger over an illness simply serves to underscore lifelong hostility or poor interpersonal relationships. In my experience, however, in most cases the following factors serve to allow patients to pass through the stage of anger:

1. A complete understanding of heart failure, including its causes, the nature of the testing required, and the treatments available.
2. Good communication with their physician, with the nursing staff, and with their support systems, that is, family, friends, or even other patients with heart failure.

3. Improvement in how they feel (even minor changes in treatment can cause significant improvement in how patients feel, and even slight improvement can alter how they feel about their disease and how willing they are to accept further information and treatment).

4. Understanding that depression is rampant in our country and that many things can contribute to depression (aging, financial stress, illness, feeling alone, and so on). Just acknowledging that you might be depressed opens the door to an improved attitude and mental health.

5. A feeling of empowerment, that is, of being in control of and responsible for the decisions in their care. Actually, all five factors are interrelated but may characterize distinct stages.

It is critical for patients to experience some improvement in how they feel. Even when a cardiologist asks me to see a patient for consideration for experimental heart failure treatment, I always carefully review all aspects of the patient's current therapy to see what modifications, albeit minor, can be performed with conventional therapies so that he or she can "feel better." This almost always restores hope to patients and their family, and serves to motivate them to let go of their anger, thus enabling them to become more accepting and understanding of their illness and more motivated to participate in their future care. Feelings of empowerment are also important. I am reminded of a patient who shared her thoughts with me when I told her that she was in control of the decision regarding heart transplantation as a treatment for her advanced form of heart failure. She reminded me that the gift availability of the donor heart was not her decision, that she had no control over the computer matchup of her need and the potential donor heart, and that some of the medical decisions would depend on her physicians' evaluation of her condition, which was, again, not in her control. However, she concluded that the bottom-line decisions were hers. She recognized that they were shared decisions but that most of life's decisions can be characterized in just this way. Thinking things through in this fashion enabled this woman, who was an interesting person and, I think, the very first patient who sat in my office for hours reading my cardiology textbooks, to maintain a feeling of empowerment. It was her struggle to take control and learn about her disease and options that started me on a different path, a path not only of delivering medical care but also of being a teacher, which is what the Latin word *doctor* means.

Let me emphasize as you read this book that there are different positions along the anger-acceptance spectrum. A patient's reaction to information and suggestions depends on his or her position. Just as I expect my patients to react differently, so too do I expect each of you to have a different reaction. However, allow yourself to accept the information and perhaps review it many times. Not all of the information will fit your individual situation, but most of it will. I hope that your journey from anger to understanding and motivation will be brief and that you will be guided by the remainder of this book. Also, I trust, as many of my patients have, that along with the passage from anger to understanding, illness to health, confusion to understanding, you also make the passage from conflict to peace.

2

The Challenge of Heart Failure

The first edition of this book was written a decade ago. I simplistically hoped when I wrote that edition that I would write the book, everyone would read it, and heart failure care would be improved, period. Okay—so I was younger and more naive. But I truly did hope that there would have been better statistics to report about heart failure a decade later. Unfortunately, the statistics remain essentially the same. Hospitals, doctors' offices, and clinics still overflow with patients who have heart failure. The good news, however, is that compared to a decade ago, more innovations and advances are available for the patient with heart failure. Those are the focus of the remainder of the book.

You are reading this book for one of many reasons. Perhaps you are one of the nearly 5 million Americans living with heart failure. Or perhaps you are among the nearly 2 million people who will be hospitalized with heart failure in the United States this year. Or one of the 10 to 15 million more who are asymptomatic (do not feel sick at all) now but are at high risk for developing heart failure in the near future. According to the readers of the first edition of this book, you may well be one of the many health professionals who treat heart failure patients every day without a complete or up-to-date understanding of what heart failure means in the 2000s and what can be done for your patients.

Will you, your spouse, or parent be one of the nearly 500,000 new cases to be diagnosed this year? Are you a sixty-five-year-old man whose heart failure was caused by years of untreated high blood pressure? Or a young woman whose diagnosis seemed to come out of the blue, with even your doctors unable to identify the cause? Have you been struck by the most common cause for hospitalization in people over the age of sixty-five? Yet heart failure affects not only the elderly but also the young (the young rock star Jim Morrison died of heart failure).

If you answered "yes" to any of the preceding questions, I have good news: You obviously are not alone! The purpose of this book is to show you that there is hope, help, and treatment for all forms of heart failure. Despite what you might have heard—and even if you heard it from your doctor—heart failure is not an automatic death sentence. It is, however, one of the most misunderstood diseases around; people regularly confuse heart failure with heart attacks. The disease's literal name is certainly disheartening; failure connotes a frightening finality. But although you may not be able to beat heart failure, you can live with it. Over the years, I have rarely seen a patient I couldn't help feel better or live longer. Heart failure patients I first met in their forties are living full, satisfying lives in their sixties. I've had senior citizens who looked as if they were at death's door make amazing progress with the right attitude and treatment. In fact, these are the keys for everyone—attitude and treatment. With the right dosages of both, you can usually improve your condition dramatically. Unfortunately, we often encounter the wrong attitudes, the wrong treatments, or both.

"YOU HAVE ONE MONTH TO LIVE"

As I will discuss later, the amazing growth in our knowledge of coronary artery disease and heart attack is what has attracted much of the interest of researchers, patients, and physicians. Although most doctors know a great deal about coronary disease, they have shown relatively little interest in heart failure. Even today, many physicians incorrectly feel there have been almost no major advances in the diagnosis and treatment of heart failure—this is true not only of general practitioners but of cardiologists as well!

Medicine has indeed made great strides in treating heart attack victims and people with clogged arteries, and doctors feel a great deal of satisfaction when they help bedridden patients become well again through angioplasty procedures, bypass operations, or other treatments. These treatments have also become relatively routine. In a nutshell, coronary disease is where the action is. Treating heart failure patients, on the other hand, has in the past not provided most doctors with the same sense of satisfaction. Surgical treatments for heart failure are the exception rather than the rule. Often, a heart failure patient lives with a great deal of uncertainty, requires frequent office visits, and experiences no major leaps of improvement from one visit to another. Slow progress is often funneled into depression or anger or frustration by the patient, the family, and even the physician. Treatment can be quite complicated, since heart failure may trigger other medical problems and result in additional complications (with the liver or kidneys, for example). Moreover, these additional problems cannot always be treated in the usual ways because of the limitations, interactions, and

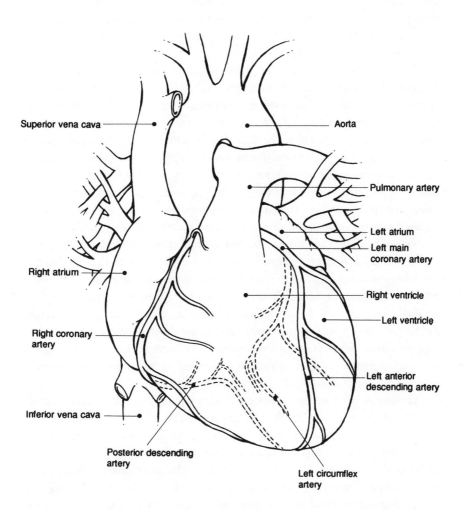

Superior vena cava

Aorta

Pulmonary artery

Left atrium

Left main
coronary artery

Right atrium

Right ventricle

Left ventricle

Right coronary
artery

Left anterior
descending artery

Inferior vena cava

Posterior descending
artery

Left circumflex
artery

This figure depicts the external structure of the normal human heart. There are four chambers: the two upper chambers (right atrium and left atrium) and two lower chambers (right ventricle and left ventricle). Blood from the upper and lower parts of the body returns to the heart via the superior vena cava and the inferior vena cava. Also shown are the major arteries, which carry the blood from the right ventricle to the lung (pulmonary artery) and from the left ventricle to the head and the rest of the body (aorta). Immediately branching off the aorta are the coronary arteries, which supply blood directly to the heart muscle. The main coronary arteries are the left main, left anterior descending, left circumflex, and the right coronary artery. (Figure courtesy of Abbott Laboratories, Abbott Park, Illinois) side-effect concerns imposed by the person's heart failure. Consequently, a percentage of doctors don't keep up with new developments in the heart failure field, preferring to focus instead on coronary disease. They labor under anachronistic notions about treatment, and some, unfortunately, inadvertently cause some patients to give up hope.

I can't tell you the number of people who have come to me and said, "My doctor told me I only have one month to live" or "My doctors say they've done all they can for me." I always tell my patients, "Doctors are not God; no one knows how long you have to live" or "I'm sure there's something I can do for you." I don't say this just to make them feel better (though it does) but because it's true. People sentenced to short-term survival often survive for many productive years! Some simply need simple medication adjustments. Others need better education and counseling on salt restriction. Someone who hasn't responded to traditional treatment may respond to an experimental procedure. Once patients realize that there are scores of things left to try and that there's a good chance at least one of them will work, their conditions often improve. This is due not only to the beneficial effect of a positive mental attitude but also to the fact that patients become more active participants in their treatment. For example, they become acutely aware of changes in how they feel and report those changes to their doctors, who then vary treatments accordingly; they watch their diet and weight carefully, making sure they stay within the doctor's recommendations; and they take their medicine in the right amounts at the right times (heart failure patients often take a number of medications, and depressed or elderly patients frequently forget to take their pills or take them at the wrong times).

Of course, none of this matters if a doctor prescribes Pill A when the patient should be receiving Pill B. This happens not because the doctor is negligent but simply because he or she is following an older, more traditional approach. For instance, digoxin is a common drug prescribed for heart failure patients that, among other things, can help the heart pump blood more strongly. This is fine for people who have a systolic problem (*systole* being the heart's contracting function, designed to squeeze blood out), but a diastolic problem (*diastole* being the relaxation of the heart between contractions) usually should *not* be treated with that drug. Digoxin causes a hard-pumping heart to pump even harder, which can have disastrous consequences, or at the very least involve the risk and expense of an additional potent heart medication.

This differentiation of heart failure into a particular type is no trivial problem. Interestingly, in patients under the age of sixty-five, about 70 percent of the time the predominant problem in heart failure is a systolic one, or a weak-pumping action of the heart; that means, however, that fully 30 percent of these patients in fact have a relaxation or diastolic problem that is causing their heart failure. Moreover, as much as 70 percent of heart failure problems in the elderly are related to poor relaxation of the heart muscle, or diastolic dysfunction. As you will see later, the problem is that treatments for these different forms of heart failure are in fact quite different; certain forms of treatment for systolic failure (poor contraction of the heart muscle) may make a person with diastolic failure (poor relaxation of the heart muscle) much worse. Because the symptoms of systolic and diastolic heart failure are often the same, it's difficult to determine the cause through cursory testing. It's easy for doctors to mistakenly jump to a conclusion and head down the wrong treatment path.

WHAT IS HEART FAILURE, ANYWAY?

The main purpose of this chapter to clear the air and define what heart failure is. As I said earlier, the term itself is ominous, but unfortunately it is one we are stuck with for now. I suspect that you are reading this book because either you, your spouse, your parent, or a close friend or relative has some form of heart failure, which is now commonly called *congestive heart failure* (CHF) but in the old days was referred to as dropsy. Recently, I gave a talk to one of our local chapters of the Mended Hearts Organization, a support group for people who primarily have cardiovascular problems. I asked for a show of hands as to how many people in the audience knew of someone, whether a spouse, relative, or neighbor, who had heart failure. Nearly two-thirds of the audience members raised their hand. I then asked for people to define heart failure. There were few accurate answers. Even worse, I recently published a research paper of a study we did. We simply asked 100 new patients who had been referred to us by other doctors, "What is heart failure?" The acceptable responses (and we took anything even close!) were less than one in three!

Now, any second-year medical student can give you the traditional definition of heart failure, namely, the inability of the cardiac function to meet the metabolic needs of the body. Unfortunately, that does not explain what heart failure truly is. I think the best way for people to think of the heart is to picture it as a pump whose job is to pump blood, which carries oxygen, or the fuel our bodies use, to the rest of the body—including arms, legs, abdomen, liver, kidneys, and brain. *Simply stated, then, heart failure is a condition in which the heart does not adequately perform its duties as a blood pump.* It is clear that a variety of malfunctions with the heart can potentially cause heart failure. I will discuss many of those in other chapters in this book. It is also obvious that if heart failure simply represents the failure of the heart to work as it should as a pump, then there may well be degrees of heart failure. And, in fact, this is true. Again, in other chapters in this book, I discuss how the kind of heart failure and its degree of severity are determined.

The main intent of this book is to demystify the very difficult and complex disease entity called heart failure and to clarify for patients, family, and friends what heart failure is really all about. I want to talk not only about what heart failure is but also about what can be done for it in both conventional and non-conventional ways. I will talk about who should be helping patients care for their heart failure, and about what patients can do to help their doctor and health care professionals care for them. I truly hope that each and every individual who reads this book will come away with a better understanding of what heart failure means today. I hope that that understanding will extend not only to patients and their families but also to other individuals in the health care field, including hospital administrators, and even, God help us, to the politicians who are going to continue to have an impact on the priorities for health care in this country.

In fact, heart failure really is a national problem because of the striking demographics of this disease. As I mentioned earlier, there are nearly 5 million people in the United States, or approximately 2 percent of our entire population, who have heart failure. And the number of cases keeps growing. The number of deaths related to heart failure alone has increased over fourfold in the last twenty years, a period in which we have waged a relatively successful war against death due to heart attack and stroke, achieving a significant decline in the mortality rate of both. In part, this increase in number of people with heart failure is related to our success in preventing patients from dying of heart attacks. As we all know, patients may survive several heart attacks and may undergo one or more bypass surgeries. Patients who survive their acute attacks may suffer damage to the heart muscle and eventually develop heart failure. Also, with the more widespread use of defibrillators, many people survive episodes of sudden death only to become symptomatic with heart failure. The other common factor underlying the major increase in the number of heart failure cases each year is the aging of our population. The largest growth group in our country is the elderly, especially those over the age of seventy-five. Information from studies tells us that the incidence of heart failure rises steadily with increasing age, so that in people over seventy-five, the incidence of heart failure is as common as one in ten!

As people age, they carry with them the cumulative subtle damages to the heart muscle brought on by coronary disease and high blood pressure; the longer one lives, the greater the likelihood of eventually developing some kind of pump problem.

The number one cause of hospitalization in the United States for people over the age of sixty-five is heart failure. Between 1973 and 1986, the number of patients discharged from a hospital with a diagnosis of heart failure more than doubled. Although hospitalization rates remained fairly stable for patients between thirty-five and fifty-four years of age, there was a substantial increase in the number of elderly patients being hospitalized, with the most significant increase being in patients over the age of seventy-four. However, the increase in the prevalence of heart failure is not simply a problem related to aging. Even when the age factor is adjusted in statistical analysis, the death rate from heart failure continues to increase twofold, suggesting that other factors operate here. Suffice it to say that heart failure is an extremely common medical problem that is increasing at an enormous rate both within the United States and throughout the world. It is a problem that taxes our medical resources and affects the daily lives of millions of men and women and their families and friends.

One of the slides I show to physicians when I talk about heart failure is labeled *Heart Failure: The Challenge for the 21st Century.* I readily acknowledge that heart failure may not surpass in importance the issue of global peace or our federal deficit, but it ranks high in terms of a major medical epidemic. We need to face this challenge at all levels in order to convert our failures into successes.

Soon I'm going to talk about some of the common causes of heart failure, what you can do to possibly prevent it, and so forth, but I do want to spend a moment discussing the statistics, or what I call the good, the bad, and the ugly of heart failure. I think these relate to questions that are on everyone's mind, and I want to clear the air as well as set the stage for the information I am about to present in this book.

Now, if one considers the statistics for even a decade ago for survival after developing heart failure, things look pretty dismal. The overall death rate from CHF within the first year of diagnosis was right around 50 percent. The good news is that today, with optimal medical treatment, that percentage has dropped below 10 percent for patients with good prognostic profiles, and it is quite reasonable to expect a five-year survival rate of well beyond 50 percent. If you are reading this book and have a very mild form of heart failure, you may find these statistics sobering, and that is one of the reasons I prefer not to quote statistics to my patients initially. These statistics tend to lump together a great many patients with a variety of different risk factors and with different forms of heart failure. There are marked differences in the outcome of heart failure, and I want to mention some of the factors that account for them.

First of all, it is commonly asked whether one sex or the other seems to have a worse prognosis with heart failure. Some studies have suggested that men have a slightly worse prognosis (60 percent versus 45 percent for the five-year mortality rate), but other studies have suggested that women have worse outcomes. I would say that, on balance, men and women seem to have the same risk of mortality. It is clear, however, that older patients do worse than younger patients, as was seen recently in a large study called the Studies of Left Ventricular Dysfunction (SOLVD), which suggested that younger patients with heart failure, ages twenty-two to fifty-five, averaged a 17 percent one-year mortality rate, whereas patients over the age of seventy-six had a 38 percent one-year mortality rate. Other risk factors, such as diabetes, atrial fibrillation (which is an irregular heartbeat of the upper chambers of the heart), and a history of smoking and alcohol consumption, also cause a worse prognosis. Interestingly, mortality in black patients seems to be about one and a half times higher than in white patients overall, but the reasons for these differences in mortality are not clear.

The problem with statistics for heart failure is that they are just that. Statistics cannot predict what will happen to you or your friend or relative. In fact, no doctor can predict how long someone with heart failure will live. There are various tools that we use to help us "guesstimate" what might happen in the future, but let me assure you that no one has a crystal ball. In the chapters ahead, I will review some of these tools, but, again, none of these are perfect. Nothing pleases me more than to see patients outlive their predicted survival statistics.

I think the lessons to be learned here are that there has been progress in the diagnosis and treatment of heart failure and that these advances have had significant impact on the overall prognosis. The flip side of the coin, however, is that with the growing prevalence of heart failure in our population we need to intensify our efforts to find new and better ways to diagnose, treat, and ultimately prevent heart failure.

HOW DO YOU GET HEART FAILURE?

As soon as your doctor diagnoses you with heart failure, you should immediately ask the $64,000 question: What caused it? Your doctor may know from your past medical history, or he or she may do a series of tests to help determine the cause. If, however, you get a vague answer like "We always see this in older folks" or "A little bit of heart failure never hurt anybody," you may already be on the wrong path (see Chapter 4).

The odds are that you'll greatly enhance the effectiveness of your treatment if you pinpoint the cause. In fact, there are many forms of heart failure that are not only treatable but also curable! The key, then, is to first determine the exact cause. The problem, of course, is that there are many causes (see Chapter 3 for a table listing the types of heart failure and their causes).

High blood pressure, or *hypertension,* is a major cause of heart failure, and there are over 60 million Americans who have it. If we could adequately treat those people, we could make a serious dent in the overall number of patients with heart failure in this country. It is estimated that even among those who know they have high blood pressure, not more than 25 percent are really treated adequately. In addressing this problem we must, I believe, put to rest two common myths.

One is that high blood pressure means the blood pressure is *always* above normal. The truth is that high blood pressure does not mean a person has an elevated blood pressure all of the time. However, the blood pressure of those who have it goes above the normal limits on occasion; the more often this occurs and the greater the extent to which their blood pressure exceeds those limits, the greater the "load" of their high blood pressure and, often, the greater the risk of damage they might sustain to their heart, kidneys, eyes, or brain. The other myth we must abandon is the notion that our blood pressure should equal 100 plus our age. This is pure hogwash. In countries where salt is not a major ingredient in the diet and exercise is more common even among the elderly, this is simply not true. With our ever-increasing elderly population, we need to educate everyone about high blood pressure even more zealously now than ever before.

The abuse of alcohol or drugs can also cause heart failure. There is a general belief, promoted by the mass media, that alcohol is beneficial for the heart (I remember clearly my beloved grandfather taking a shot of whiskey daily before meals until he died in his ninth decade of life). However, although there is some evidence that limited alcohol may be helpful in preventing some forms of heart problems related to the coronary arteries, there is clear evidence that alcohol is a definite toxin, or damaging substance, to the heart muscle. Therefore, whether a person's heart failure was caused by years of alcohol abuse or not, I recommend that alcohol be avoided forever. I usually tell my patients that they may enjoy a single alcoholic beverage on Christmas, their wedding anniversary, or their birthday—but that's it. When they ask about once a month and then once a week, or even two or three times a week, I usually suspect that they may in fact have an alcohol problem. I forbid my patients to have alcohol at all and help those who cannot comply to seek counseling.

Over the past several years the role of alcohol for patients with heart failure continues to be debated. Indeed, some of my colleagues point to data that suggests that patients who drink moderately may not do any worse when they were studied in large clinical trials. I acknowledge the data but my personal observation and opinion is that patients who cannot exert their power of self-control over alcohol (or salt or fluids, and so forth) are not likely to be as successful as they can. And so if you see me as your doctor, plan on not drinking alcohol.

Other causes of heart failure include the following: blocked heart arteries, even with no history of a heart attack (coronary artery disease); heart attack, which may be a "silent" one the patient isn't aware of; inflammation of the heart muscle, which may accompany a simple cold or flulike illness and is often caused by a virus that settles in the heart muscle; narrowed or leaky heart valves, which can result from rheumatic fever, congenital problems, or even an aging process; numerous blood transfusions (the repeated transfusions required because of a genetic or acquired blood problem can create iron buildup in the heart); pregnancy (see Chapter 15); and AIDS, or acquired immunodeficiency syndrome (see Chapter 15).

Doctors may tell their patients that the cause of their heart failure is *idiopathic dilated cardiomyopathy*. What this scientific-sounding phrase really means is "We don't know what caused your heart muscle to weaken." This is an especially troublesome situation because doctors are unable to tie treatment to a specific cause. I will refer to these different causes of heart failure later, but first I will address a common question, namely, "How can I lessen my risk of developing heart failure?"

PREVENTION

Because of heart failure's many causes, preventive measures are so far only partially effective. Nevertheless, the following motto, which I recently shared with the audience at a lecture on geriatric heart failure, is useful: "The cure for heart failure in the elderly is prevention of cardiovascular disease in the young." Certainly, you should do everything possible to lower high blood pressure and to follow the commonsense advice about not smoking, watching your weight and cholesterol levels, and exercising. Unfortunately, all these steps may not guarantee that you will avoid heart failure. A virus can strike anyone, regardless of how healthy he or she might be. Or you may be the victim of a genetic predisposition to heart failure, or you may have required a series of blood transfusions related to another medical problem, for example, sickle-cell anemia.

In fact, we currently do a much better job preventing other forms of heart disease. Ironically, our preventive success with other heart diseases has funneled an increasing number of people into the heart failure category. The odds are that you've been hearing about more and more people who have been told they have heart failure. Why? Because we've become so proficient at helping people survive heart attacks with the use of clot-busting drugs and devices and surgery. The people who survive one or more heart attacks or have bypass surgery (which is sometimes done even two or three times) are the ones who eventually develop weakened hearts that lead to heart failure. We've statistically increased the chances of the average person falling victim to heart failure; having found effective treatments for many forms of heart disease, cancer, diabetes, and so on, we've simply allowed people to avoid one disease in favor of another. There's nothing wrong with this. If anything, it emphasizes our growing need to focus not only on doing what we can to prevent heart failure but also on doing everything we can as early as possible to determine if we have it.

As I conclude this section on prevention I must share with you some exciting news that truly is hot off the press. As I mentioned in the last edition, a new blood test called BNP (B-type natriuretic peptide, see the next chapter on diagnosis) has recently become available. Working with this test we realized that the test might detect some weakness of the heart muscle even before a person had any signs or symptoms. However, since most doctors are currently using the BNP level to detect the degree of heart muscle weakness a person already diagnosed with heart failure might have, we saw the opportunity to detect early heart failure in a group of patients who had risk factors for heart failure but who did not yet have the disease. Therefore we recently held what we believe are the very first screening clinics for heart failure. We invited patients who had risk factors for heart failure such as high blood pressure, diabetes mellitus, coronary artery disease, family history, and so on to come in and answer some questions and get a BNP level drawn. None of these patients were aware or ever told they might have heart failure. To our surprise, over 10 percent of these patients did indeed have an elevated BNP level; early follow-up of these patients suggests that often with the aid of the elevated BNP level their doctors did perform confirmatory tests and many did show early heart failure. Other had appropriate heart failure medications added.

So prevention of heart failure seems even more closely within our grasp than ever before. I suspect that the BNP blood test will be more widely applied in the years ahead and that it will allow patients and doctors to get an enormous jump on the early detection and the prevention of heart failure for millions.

THE ASYMPTOMATIC MANY

The best time to begin treatment for heart failure is before you know you have it. If that seems like a paradox, consider the fact that many people have heart failure for years and aren't aware of it. Just as we can function with one kidney or one lung, we can often function with our heart working at 50 percent of its normal capacity. I always tell my patients that the good Lord gives us a little extra of everything and that it's not how much heart muscle we have but how efficiently we use it. Although the onset of heart failure can be sudden and can create the same kind of instant trauma as a heart attack, it usually progresses insidiously over a long period of time. During that progression, your heart becomes weaker and weaker, though you feel perfectly fine. It is during that period, often called the "asymptomatic period" or the "preclinical" era, that patients quietly but insidiously use up the reserve that the body naturally has. When symptoms finally surface, you've already passed an important window of opportunity—the early stages of the disease, which are the optimal treatment time.

We know that if you treat people when they're asymptomatic, the number of times they'll be hospitalized is fewer, the progression of the disease is slower, and the overall survival rate may be higher. Even though you're asymptomatic, you can determine if you're at high risk for heart failure by asking yourself the following questions:

- Have you ever had a heart attack?
- Have you ever had any infection of the heart or a previous inflammation around the heart?
- Do you have a heart murmur?
- Are you overweight?
- Do you have high blood pressure?
- Are you a heavy drinker, smoker, or drug abuser?
- Do you have diabetes?
- Do you have a family history of heart failure? (Prevailing medical opinion used to be that there is no correlation between heart failure and family history; in the face of mounting evidence to the contrary, that opinion is now changing.)

If you answered "yes" to any of these questions, you're at high risk; the more "yes" answers, the higher the risk.

Go to your doctor and tell him or her of your concerns. Depending on many things, including your history and the signs and symptoms you have, your doctor may perform a variety of tests and procedures aimed at determining if you have heart failure and, if so, what form of heart failure you have and what your current status is. These are discussed in Chapter 3.

TELLTALE SIGNS

After the asymptomatic stage is the stage in which a person receives early warning signs of heart failure. Again, the faster the following signs are heeded, the better the prognosis:

- Shortness of breath (during activities, shortly after lying down in bed at night, or both)
- Fatigue (may start slowly—just being more tired after work)
- Chest pains (in chest, back, neck, throat, arms, pit of stomach, and so on)
- Swollen feet (may start at the end of the day)
- Weight gain or loss
- Changes in appetite
- Inability to shake a cold or other relatively minor illness

If you have one or more of these signs, the underlying cause could be any one of a host of things besides heart failure. To enable you to compare your symptoms with theirs, here are some of the descriptions heart failure patients commonly use to express their physical problems: They notice that they can no longer participate in a regular activity or sport without feeling fatigued or short of breath. For instance, golfers complain that they used to play eighteen holes without a problem and now are very tired after nine holes. Some people say they now have to sit down and rest after cleaning one room of the house, whereas before they could clean all the rooms without feeling tired. Whether the activity is shoveling snow or walking up the stairs, in all the cases, people find that they can no longer do what they once did with ease. In many instances, they rationalize the problem rather than consult a doctor. Typically, they attribute their fatigue or shortness of breath to getting older, weight gain, or being out of shape.

ARE YOU RECEIVING
THE RIGHT TREATMENT?

Early treatment is important for many reasons, not the least of which is its potential to control heart failure's impact on the other parts of the body. Since the body is an interactive system, the heart's failure affects other parts of that system, including the lungs, kidneys, liver, brain, and muscles. For example, heart failure often precipitates kidney failure, since an insufficient amount of blood is being pumped to those organs; this process is usually insidious but may be hastened by underlying kidney damage from high blood pressure or diabetes. Similarly, untreated heart failure leads to shortness of breath, which in turn makes people inactive and homebound, which leads to a greatly deconditioned state, which usually makes the person even more symptomatic.

If, however, heart failure is treated at an early stage, the damage can be postponed and limited. You may be able to postpone kidney damage indefinitely or for years, instead of for months, and you may be able to avoid the poor muscle tone that could turn you into an invalid.

Even if you don't seek medical help in the early stages of the disease, your prospects are probably better than you think. As I mentioned before, not so long ago, at least 50 percent of the people diagnosed with heart failure died within a year of diagnosis. Today, with optimal treatment, that percentage has decreased to below 10 percent for many people—those with good prognostic profiles.

More important, I feel, is the fact that heart failure patients are feeling better and doing more than ever before. Though it's difficult to quantify quality-of-life issues, I've seen a dramatic turnaround in this area: I have patients who formerly would have been bedridden and now go on ski trips, work regular jobs, and live well-rounded lives. With today's approaches and treatments for heart failure, most patients should be able to make some progress toward feeling better and doing more. If a person has been on a steady decline since being diagnosed with heart failure, he or she may need attention to the typical problem areas discussed in the following paragraphs.

TREATING THE GENERAL SYMPTOMS, NOT THE SPECIFIC CAUSE

There's a standard regimen of drugs and other treatments that doctors prescribe for heart failure patients. This prescription is fine for a significant percentage of patients but not for a sizable minority. For instance, heart failure can be caused by inflammation of the heart muscle. If a doctor fails to do a heart biopsy, he or she will not learn that this is the problem in a given case and will not prescribe treatment specific to this cause. Although treatment for this kind of heart problem remains controversial, many experts think that using certain anti-inflammatory drugs can alter the destructive heart process. Or the doctor might not realize that the patient's condition is a result of a silent heart attack, that the patient has coronary problems that require different medications from the ones he or she has been prescribing. It is vitally important for doctors to pinpoint the causes of heart failure in their patients so that they can provide optimal treatment.

FALSE ASSUMPTIONS ABOUT HEART FAILURE

Clearly, when heart failure has been going on for ten years or more, it's more difficult to reverse all the damage. Someone who has heart failure due to twenty-five years of severe high blood pressure, for instance, probably has a permanently weakened heart muscle. This person may be helped but probably will never regain complete heart function. But when heart failure occurs suddenly—for example, when it is caused by a virus or is associated with an irregular heartbeat or a pregnancy in a previously healthy woman—it's quite possible to help the patient recover completely. But that won't happen if you're a short-term heart failure patient who's treated like a long-term one. The key to success: Your doctor must recognize that the disease has been relatively brief, pinpoint the cause, and tailor the treatment accordingly.

NO REEVALUATION

Heart function doesn't become static or predictable when a person has heart failure; it's always getting worse or getting better. When doctors first diagnose heart failure patients, they may grade their condition on one or more "scales" to determine how serious their heart failure may be. They may grade symptoms on a one to four scale (four being the worst). This is called the New York Heart Association Functional Class and is commonly used to assess a person's symptoms. (Also see Chapter 3.) Another gradation of the heart muscle function is an ejection fraction scale of 0 to 50 percent (0 percent being the worst). The ejection fraction tells your doctor how much blood the heart pumps with each beat and also contributes to a person's overall prognosis in general.

These scales can be monitored regularly to detect changes in heart function and to make sure that patients continue to receive treatment that is appropriate. If their condition becomes worse, treatment is changed or intensified. If their condition improves, certain therapies can be eliminated (which may improve the way patients feel even more).

A BIG BAG OF TRICKS

In many ways, heart failure is a highly individualized disease. The treatment that's right for one person might be wrong for someone else. A slight change in therapy might make all the difference in the world. Fortunately, doctors are becoming more adept at tailoring treatments to patients. We have a big bag of tricks to choose from, some simple and some complex. Some of the things you'll find in that bag are the following:

- Dietary restriction of salt and fluids
- Changing the types of drugs patients are receiving
- Changing the drug dosages
- Using experimental drugs
- Heart transplants
- Experimental surgeries and devices
- Artificial hearts

Though I'll discuss these and other therapies in greater detail in later chapters, let me address a few issues that this list raises.

Many patients often ask, "Why can't I get a heart transplant? My neighbor had one, and it was like a miracle." Heart transplants *can* have miraculous effects. Certainly, the idea of exchanging an old, failing heart for a young, healthy one is appealing. But heart transplants aren't for everyone. Generally, age sixty-five is the cutoff for transplants. In addition, people with other medical problems are usually not good transplant candidates (for example, the drugs given to patients after the transplant to suppress immune systems can play havoc with insulin-dependent diabetes). Third, the number of donors is limited; there are only about 3,000 transplants done annually (see Chapter 9).

Then, what about an artificial heart? Again, the idea is appealing, but reality hasn't yet caught up with the ideal. In most instances, artificial hearts are used as "bridges" to transplants; that is, they sustain a patient until a donor heart is available. Although a number of improvements in artificial hearts have been made—there are now small, internally implanted models that don't require huge external machines—they aren't, as of yet, the panacea people initially hoped they would be. However, they remain one of the great hopes of the future (see Chapter 17).

A lot of attention has been given to some of the newer surgical techniques available for heart failure (see also Chapter 12). Among these are aggressive use of mitral valve repair and replacement, partial left ventricular ventriculectomy, and what I consider one of the more promising experimental surgeries, called a cardiac restraint device. This involves taking a device (such as an Acorn device) and wrapping it around a weak heart. These devices seem to not only limit the progressive increase in heart size but also allow the heart to begin to shrink back toward a normal size. Work is now being done to use special materials to make these devices work better (Acorn or Paracor devices). Also, soon these devices will be able to be placed with minimally invasive surgery. One of the great advantages this technique has over transplantation is that there's no danger of rejection.

For now, the best treatments generally involve drugs, dietary restrictions, and exercise. However, mechanical devices, pacemakers, and surgical techniques are quickly emerging as important additive measures. Tremendous strides in this area have been made, creating new, more effective medications with fewer side effects, and learning how to use them in combination with others to make heart failure patients feel better and live longer. There are many experimental drugs, some of which will probably enable us to take the next great step forward in our fight against heart failure.

HOW DO YOU DEFINE SUCCESS?

The definition of success in treating heart failure varies and depends on the patient's goals, age, and condition. All patients with heart failure want to feel better and be able to do more. The elderly may have other goals, such as being less dependent on family or neighbors or being able to attend a granddaughter's wedding. For a younger person, an important goal may be being able to get back to work. Certainly, long-term survival is a bigger issue for the nineteen-year-old than for the ninety-year-old. Some patients may want to find out more about what heart failure is and how they can help themselves more.

The pages that follow will help patients achieve these objectives. Success is possible. Though no magic cure exists, it is important for patients to know that numerous options are available that can make a significant difference in treatment effectiveness. Time and again, I've seen heart failure patients who have given up hope prematurely, who have limited their activities unnecessarily, who have suffered needlessly, and who have been denied optimum treatment.

THE IMPORTANCE OF BEING OPTIMISTIC

More than most diseases, heart failure demands patient participation. Patients can impact their treatment by being acute observers of their condition, by communicating crucial information to their doctor, by following the regimen he or she recommends, and by being optimistic. The last suggestion may sound Pollyannaish, but I've found that optimistic heart failure patients do far better than pessimistic ones. Too often, a heart failure diagnosis becomes a self-fulfilling prophecy: Sure that every day is their last, people start acting like they're doomed and treat their bodies like fragile antiques.

Recently, at the request of a cardiologist, I saw a seventy-year-old woman with heart failure. Her doctor said she was "terribly sick," had been in and out of the hospital, and was now receiving treatments at home. He added that it was difficult for him to convince her and her family to come to my outpatient center to see me; the patient was afraid to be moved and wondered if it was worth the effort. Finally, she agreed to come in, but her family insisted that she come by ambulance.

After her arrival by ambulance, the patient was brought into my waiting room on a stretcher, with oxygen running, and a somewhat nervous receptionist called me to say that my patient had arrived. I examined the patient and found that she was in relatively good shape, that her heart was fairly strong, and that the reason her cardiologist had said she was terribly sick was related to secondary problems that were eminently treatable. I spent ninety minutes with the patient explaining what I had found and the adjustments in treatment that should be made. Finally, I told her that there was no reason for her to be on the stretcher, that she did not need the oxygen, and that she could help herself by beginning to walk more and more each day. I had her walk around the room, and she was both amazed and delighted that she could do so. Since her son was in the waiting room, I suggested to her that she walk out of my office on her own two legs to meet him, which she did.

A few minutes later another doctor came in, shaking his head. I asked him what was the matter. "The receptionist," he said, "just told me something that I thought you'd appreciate. She said, 'I heard Dr. Silver was good, but I've never seen anything like that. A woman comes in almost comatose on a stretcher, with oxygen, and a little while later she walks out with a bounce in her step and a smile on her face.'"

Certainly, I hope this book helps you live longer. But just as important, I hope it puts a bounce in your step and a smile on your face as you find success with heart failure.

3

Evaluating Your Condition

Many heart failure patients possess either erroneous, vague, or even more often, *no* information about their condition. That is why I wrote this book. I did not need to do a research study to prove this fact to myself. Nonetheless, since our world of medicine has become "evidence-based," which means you don't really know something unless you've scientifically measured it, I did such a study, and it was published in the medical journal *Congestive Heart Failure.* Basically, in this study we asked 100 patients who were having their first visit with me several questions. Now, bear in mind that all these patients had seen another doctor before coming to see me; 89 percent of them had also been to see another cardiologist, and 46 percent had seen two or more cardiologists before their visit with me. At their visit, we asked them the following questions:

1. *What is heart failure?*

On this question we took almost anything as a correct answer, such as "The heart is weak," "The pump's no good," "The muscle has been damaged," and so on.

2. *Have you ever been told to restrict your sodium intake? If you have, do you follow a restricted sodium diet?*

The idea here was to see if anywhere along the line of their treatment for heart failure, including a referral to a heart failure and heart transplant specialist, anyone had ever impressed upon them the need to reduce the salt intake in their diets; all of these patients, by the way, were already on potent diuretics (water pills), whose job is to get rid of excess fluid and salt in the body.

3.   *Have you ever been told to restrict your fluid intake? If you have, do you follow a fluid restricted diet?*

Same idea here—to see if they had the necessary information to help themselves with their heart failure. All of these patients, by the way, were already on potent diuretics (water pills).

4.   *Were you ever told to weigh yourself daily? If so, do you do it?*

As you will read later in this book, one of the most important things you can do is to monitor your own body weight. This is important for many reasons, but one of them is to have an early warning system to detect fluid accumulation, so that it can be properly treated. We asked this question to see if this group of patients had ever heard this notion before coming to see us.

&

The results are, at the least, disconcerting. I realized after analyzing the results that just because a person could not tell you that he or she had never heard of a salt or fluid restriction it didn't mean that somewhere along the line it had never been mentioned; it simply meant that a single instruction, not repeated often and without a person being told the "why" of it, won't be incorporated into a daily habit, especially in a person who has a serious illness with many other worries on his or her mind.

Well, here are the answers to the questions:

Question	Adequate response (%)	Inadequate response (%)
What is CHF?	33	67
Told of sodium?	72	28
Limits sodium?	67	33
Told of fluid?	18	72
Limits fluid?	12	88
Told to weigh?	11	89
Actually weighs?	9	91

As you can see, my deepest concerns were confirmed in this study. Again, this did not tell me that these patients *never* were told things about heart failure, but rather that if they were told, it didn't or couldn't sink in. The latter could be due to so many other problems associated with heart failure, such as advanced age, previous strokes, poor blood flow to the brain, effects of medication, and so forth. The remarkable feature of the study, however, is that when patients did recall being told something about their heart failure, such as restricting sodium or weighing daily, most actually did so (93 percent and 82 percent, respectively).

This is truly the reason I wrote this book in the first place. Everyone learns differently; some learn by hearing information, others by reading it. Most of us usually need to hear or see instructions repeated several times or have a guide to go back and assure ourselves of the correct answer. This book, I hope, will be that reference guidebook for patients and their families.

Now, I mentioned my belief that most patients do not really know enough about some of the basics of heart failure, and I believe (and know) that other misconceptions and inaccuracies abound, for most patients not only underestimate or overestimate the seriousness of their condition, but also they often don't know the specific cause of their heart failure and don't comprehend how it developed and how it evolved.

We doctors are to blame, in part, for this situation. For too long, we've lumped all heart failure patients into the same category. We don't admit that heart failure is a relatively unexplored medical territory, and instead of telling patients we don't know, we sometimes make unfounded guesses and inadvertently communicate the wrong information. Even today, some physicians betray their fatalistic attitudes about the disease, sending false messages to patients that there is no help or hope.

Considering the advances we've made in heart failure diagnosis and treatment, there is no reason for doctors to continue these practices. For both psychological and treatment reasons, people need an accurate assessment of where they stand as heart failure patients. Psychologically, patients require accurate information to deal with their disease; sometimes, just knowing what caused it can remove some of their anxiety. I truly believe that people want to know the details. From a treatment perspective, patients benefit from knowing the cause, type, and stage of their heart failure; we're in a much better position to improve patients' quality of life and help them battle the disease if they are informed participants in their treatment.

I will examine several classification systems for heart failure and the diagnostic methods available to patients, and see what they can reveal about an individual's condition.

CLASSIFICATION OF HEART FAILURE

Just recently the American College of Cardiology (ACC) and the American Heart Association (AHA) updated and published their well-respected guidelines for the diagnosis and treatment of heart failure. I had the privilege to serve on this task force and help rewrite the current guidelines. One of the first things we felt important to change was the perspective on how everyone viewed heart failure. We felt there was not enough attention being given to the early stages of heart failure. Therefore, what you will see below reflects an older and still useful classification referred to as the New York Heart Association, or NYHA class. It is still commonly used (I use it each time I see a patient), but its only flaw is that if a patient has a worse class one day and then later improves slightly to a better class, the better class may tend to give the patient *and* the doctor a false sense of security that indeed everything is okay. Although this book is certainly about help and hope, a key point to be made is that once you do have symptoms of heart failure you are in a precarious position and you need to get and maintain the best health care possible.

Following the NYHA class I give you the newest stages of heart failure that appear in the guidelines.

A classification system based on patient symptoms was developed years ago. Called the New York Heart Association Functional Classification, it divides heart patients into four categories:

Functional Class I: Asymptomatic; patient is not short of breath or fatigued with any activity.

Functional Class II: Patient is short of breath or fatigued after moderate activity (such as climbing two flights of stairs, golfing nine holes, or carrying a load of wash up from the basement).

Functional Class III: Patient is short of breath or fatigued even after very mild exertion (such as walking across the house or up half a flight of stairs).

Functional Class IV: Patient is exhausted, short of breath, or fatigued when just sitting still or lying down in bed.

Data exist that suggest that even a simple classification like this can help determine how a heart failure patient may do in the future, but relatively few physicians apply this functional classification system on a routine basis. This I consider a serious problem. Although even I find the classification faulty, I am constantly reminded of its use. What I mean by this is that there is, on occasion, a patient who defies classification, for example, individuals who during the day can climb stairs, mow the lawn, and so on, but who at night have episodes of awakening to catch their breath. During the day they may be a NYHA Functional Class I yet a Functional Class IV at night. This may be due to angina at night, too much fluid taken in the evening hours, and so on, and therefore may make the classification seem absurd by having the entire range of prognosis in the same patient. (Obviously, here, we would try and remedy the night situation so that all of the person's symptoms fit into a single NYHA functional classification.)

On the other hand, a research fellow from another university came to spend some time working with me, and we set about analyzing the best early predictors for death or the need for a heart transplant in a large group of our patients. I had anticipated several other, more complicated features to best predict the outcome and we were both surprised to see that the NYHA Functional Classification was the quickest and simplest tool. Therefore, I encourage you and your doctors to use it.

Stages of Heart Failure (a newer classification system) from ACC/AHA Guidelines

Stage A. Patients who are at increased risk for developing heart failure due to associated medical conditions (such as hypertension, coronary artery disease, or diabetes mellitus).

Heart structure and function is not yet affected

Potential therapies: Treatment of hypertension, smoking cessation, and weight loss; ACE inhibitors in appropriate patients

Stage B. Patients who have abnormal heart structure and/or function but who have not manifested signs or symptoms.

Heart structure and function: abnormal

Potential therapies: Same, plus ACE inhibitors and beta-blockers in all appropriate patients

Stage C. Patients with symptomatic heart failure. These patients indeed have advanced heart failure. Note that development of signs and symptoms occurs as late phenomena after significant perturbation of many homeostatic mechanisms and consumption of large cardiac reserves.

Heart structure and function: abnormal

Potential therapies: Same, plus ACE inhibitors, beta-blockers as well as digoxin and diuretics in most patients. Also, coronary revascularization and repair of mitral regurgitation in selected patients

Stage D. Patients with extremely advanced heart failure.

Heart structure and function: extremely abnormal

Potential therapies: Same, consideration of advanced therapies including investigational therapies, as well as end-of-life counseling and hospice.

(ACE = Angiotensin converting enzyme)

One of the important aspects of these stages is that it represents a forward progression and once someone has advanced to one stage they can never go back to an earlier stage—the lesson again is—*you can never go back*—so work to maintain your health!

DIAGNOSTIC TESTS

Ejection Fraction

One of the most important measurements we take, which serves both as a baseline measurement and as a means of following a person's progress, is of the *ejection fraction,* which is the amount of blood the heart ejects or pumps with each contraction. The normal ejection fraction for the left side of the heart is approximately 50–60 percent, and it is 45–55 percent for the right side. Obviously, there is a gradation, but anything below 25 percent suggests an unfavorable prognosis. A measurement of about 35 percent or higher offers a much better prognosis for long-term survival. (Note, however, that this is quite variable: Someone at 37 percent may not do as well as someone at 15 or 20 percent!)

Three methods exist for measuring ejection fractions, and each makes the measurement differently. To get more information and enhance the reliability of the diagnosis, a doctor may use two or more of the methods.

When these tests are complete, patients can be fairly certain of the accuracy of both the left and right ventricle ejection fractions. If your doctor fails to perform one or more of these measurements, you should ask why, so that you can understand how your doctor is evaluating your degree and type of heart failure.

Cardiac Catheterization. In *cardiac catheterization* (left ventricular angiogram), contrast material or dye is injected into the left ventricle of the heart, which allows the measurement of the shape and volume of the heart. On the plus side, this method provides a relatively accurate measurement of the ejection fraction by calculating the volume of blood in the heart just before the heart squeezes, and the volume after the heart has squeezed out all it can with a single beat. On the minus side, it's an invasive measure that carries a small degree of risk.

MUGA Test. In a *MUGA* (multiple gated acquisition) *test,* or *RNA* (radionuclide angiogram), a small dose of radioactive material is injected into the bloodstream and a scanning machine then tracks this material, revealing how much blood is ejected from the heart, much like a cardiac catheterization. One of the best attributes of this test is that, with certain modifications, and if requested by the doctor, it can also measure the ejection fraction of the right ventricle. Typically, the left ejection fraction receives more attention, since the majority of heart failure patients have problems there, but we've found that the right ejection fraction is often a good predictor of a patient's survival and that it complements rather than duplicates the prediction made by the left ejection fraction.

Echocardiogram. The *echocardiogram,* another noninvasive procedure, bounces sound waves off the heart to provide an ejection fraction reading (among other important measurements of the heart). Though it's helpful in revealing enlarged hearts and in determining whether the problem is primarily diastolic or systolic, it may not always provide good visualization, since the echo beam has to pass through various structures in the chest. Also, it can over- or underestimate the ejection fraction. However, if a good heart image is obtained, this is a very useful test, since it can often give good information about heart valves, the sac that envelops the heart, called the pericardium, and even what the pressures are within the heart and lungs—all noninvasively!

Treadmill Testing and Cardiopulmonary Exercise Testing

Since one of the most common manifestations of heart failure is shortness of breath as people move about or exert themselves, one of the best ways to see how symptomatic they really are is to put them on a treadmill and have them exercise. This, of course, has been done for years to see if people with coronary artery disease develop chest pain or changes in their electrocardiogram. Also, treadmills are used to make sure the drugs we use to treat coronary artery disease or high blood pressure are working.

One of the surprising facts to emerge from exercise testing with heart failure patients, however, is that there is very little relationship between the number of seconds or minutes a person with heart failure can walk on the treadmill and his or her overall survival. Nonetheless, many patients with heart failure commonly get a treadmill test, and this may be an important part of the screening process to determine the cause of the heart failure and to get a rough idea of how symptomatic an individual is. Treadmill tests are often combined with other procedures that take a picture of the blood flow to the heart, such as a thallium scan.

Aware of the limitations of the regular treadmill in terms of prognostic ability, doctors have increasingly turned their attention to a more specific way of looking at how the heart and lungs work together to provide blood and oxygen to the remainder of the body. This is yet another form of exercise test, which I will describe in just a moment. First, let me review an important concept.

As I mentioned before, we all have a little extra heart function, so people can have their ejection fractions drop down to half of normal and may still not notice any change whatsoever at rest or with minimal activity. However, since one of the key symptoms of heart failure is exercise intolerance, it is when people start to do things—walk, work, exercise—that they notice difficulties. Because the measurements of ejection fraction are done at rest, they often give little useful information about how limited a person may be with exercise. (Sometimes, we can do exercise MUGAs or exercise echocardiograms to get this information.) Also, since the heart must pump blood through an extensive network of blood vessels to get it to the muscles to do the work of walking, lifting, and so on, it is important to test how the heart, lungs, blood vessels, and muscles all work together during exercise to really determine how patients use what they have in terms of heart function. ("It's not what you have but how you use it," I often tell patients.) One of the best ways we can do that is with a cardiopulmonary exercise test (CPX), which checks the heart's and lungs' ability to deliver blood and oxygen to muscles. By measuring peak oxygen consumption, which reflects the maximal amount of blood the heart can pump to the tissues, we can obtain an accurate and reproducible measure of a heart patient's condition. The big problem with this measurement is that the particular exercise testing equipment needed for it isn't widely available. Aside from a few heart failure specialists and universities, most doctors don't have access to this equipment. Until cardiopulmonary testing equipment becomes more readily available, this valuable test cannot be routinely offered to many patients.

There are other exercise measurements available; many physicians are currently using a six-minute walk test (the ground the patient can cover in a total of six minutes) to help fill the gap when CPX testing cannot be done. This seems to have some proven reliability for heart failure patients. I feel, however, that the CPX is the superior measurement.

Stress Hormone Test

A variety of chemicals or hormones are produced by the body as a result of damage to the heart muscle. Over the last decade, we have gained a tremendous amount of knowledge about these substances, which we call neurohormones. A neurohormone means a hormone produced by the brain—which was originally thought to be where these hormones originated and where many of them were discovered.

However, as we learned more, we discovered several interesting facts, including the following:

- The hormones are produced everywhere in the body, including the heart itself and the lining of the blood vessels.
- Not only are the substances present in increased quantity in the blood in patients with heart failure, but also the level or degree of elevation in the blood can help determine a patient's prognosis.

Usually, these hormones are not only "present" in the blood but they also are part of a process that allows the substances to help contribute to the heart muscle's deterioration. Therefore, these neurohormones are not only "markers" or tags for the extent of the disease but they also contribute to the progression and process.

Perhaps one of the biggest advances in heart failure comes from regarding the usefulness and the availability of one of these neurohormones. I am referring to B-type natriuretic hormone, or BNP. When I wrote the last edition of this book I began to refer to the little information that was available about BNP. At that time it seemed like BNP was going to be a helpful marker of a person's heart failure. Well, two major advances have occurred that, in my mind, make BNP one of the most important neurohormones to check. First of all, when I last wrote, BNP was an interesting test but one that had to be sent to an outside laboratory (I used to send mine to the Mayo Clinic labs; this usually meant at least a seven- to ten-day period before any results were available). Recently, a company call Biosite has introduced an assay for BNP that is extremely reliable and can be done right away. Our hospital was the first one to use this BNP assay in Illinois but now many more hospitals are using the Biosite test and hopefully this will become a common and readily available test for checking on a patient with heart failure. The other useful information is that we have learned that the BNP level itself is reliable and reproducible. Further, the level of the BNP in the blood can help us make decisions about whether someone needs to be admitted into the hospital and the adequacy of their medications, as well as distinguish whether symptoms and signs such as shortness of breath and leg edema likely stem from their heart failure or are unrelated—this is so important!

Further, as I discuss later, we have also used BNP to help detect people who are at risk but have no signs or symptoms of heart failure at a very, very early stage. This has given us a useful step closer to our goal of heart failure prevention.

Suffice it to say that I am personally excited about having BNP as a marker for heart failure and it has made a big impact on my patients.

Listed below are some of the neurohormones that are available that many heart failure specialists look at to determine a person's status and degree of heart failure. These include the following:

- *Atrial naturetic peptide (ANP):* Originally found in the upper chambers of the heart, hence the name atrial, this can be found in many tissues and is elevated in heart failure.
- *B-type natriuretic peptide (BNP):* As above. In fact these hormones, because they can cause diuresis (help get rid of fluid), naturesis (help get rid of salt), and vasodilatation are becoming more widely used to treat

heart failure patients. Also, these neurohormones can easily be assayed or tested to determine a person's degree of heart failure.

- *Renin:* A hormone secreted from the kidney in response to what the kidneys perceive as impaired blood flow. This hormone can cause excessive production of other damaging hormones, including angiotensin II.

- *Angiotensin II (or AII):* A potent hormone that causes excessive constriction or narrowing of the blood vessels, which can make the blood pressure rise and make the heart work harder. Also, AII can cause abnormal amounts of scar tissue to form in the heart and around the blood vessels, as well as directly damage the heart muscle more.

- *Tumor necrosis factor alpha (TNF alpha):* A fascinating hormone first found to be secreted by cancer cells. This hormone has profound effects on making the heart weaker as well as being capable of causing many of the signs and symptoms of heart failure, including muscle weakness and wasting, poor appetite, fatigue, and so on.

- *Catecholamines:* These stress hormones are normally present in our bodies and are responsible for the "flight or fight" reaction during stressful periods. However, with even minor damage to the heart muscle, these chemicals are poured out into the bloodstream on a constant basis and can cause many effects, including more constriction of the blood vessels, which makes the heart work harder, as well as causing direct damage to the heart muscle. In addition, these hormones can cause excessive release of other hormones that can add to the damage and propagate the entire downhill course for a patient.

As I said, we can draw a blood test and easily measure and monitor these levels, and I find them very important pieces of the puzzle. Since they are often elevated long before a person "feels" sick, they can serve as early warning devices. In fact, I believe that some form of neurohormone measurement will be part of how we screen patients for heart failure in the future.

As I mentioned earlier, the catecholamines are one of the first discovered neurohormones to play a role in heart failure prognosis and progression, and I do measure one of the catecholamines in most patients on a regular basis. Aside from the BNP test the other one I often perform is the plasma norepinephrine level. A simple blood test will reveal your stress hormone, or plasma norepinephrine, level. This hormone, which is normally released during periods of stress, helps you cope with powerful emotions by causing the heart to pump stronger and faster. When your heart muscle weakens, your body senses that loss of strength and your stress hormone level goes up and stays up. Years ago, heart failure expert Dr. Jay Cohn conducted a study that revealed that patients with high plasma norepinephrine levels had a markedly greater chance (80 percent) of dying within two years than patients with near-normal levels, the two-year mortality rate dipping down to less than 20 percent for patients with a normal level. The stress hormone test remains one of the important prognostic indicators or "guesstimators" for heart failure.

Other Measurements of Neurohormones

Like the plasma norepinephrine level, which is a reflection of a chemical appearing in the blood as a result of a complicated and sensitive bodily reaction to impaired heart function, there are many, many more such reactions occurring in the body. Indeed, the discovery of this chemical in the blood of patients has made a major impact on our understanding of how heart failure develops and progresses. We initially simply "discovered" norepinephrine in the blood and only later related its presence to survival, and even later to its role in the propagation and progression of the failing heart. We now know, for example, that the norepinephrine chemical actually can damage heart muscle cells and lead to the progression of heart failure. That is why so many of the drugs we think may be beneficial in heart failure actually seem to attenuate or diminish the production of the norepinephrine, or at least lower its level in the blood.

Since the discovery of norepinephrine in the blood, many other "hormones," as well as what are now called "cytokines," have been discovered either to play an important role in heart failure development and progression or in some cases are deficient in the blood of patients who have heart failure.

To me, one of the most interesting discussions going on in heart failure diagnosis and treatment surrounds the role of cytokines. Cytokines are potent chemicals produced by cells and are almost everywhere in the body. Usually, they repair injury to cells and get the process going. They can initiate a bodily response and turn on the immune system. This is usually intended to be a good thing, or what we call preserving "homeostasis." We have discovered that often these "normal" responses turn out to be exaggerated and potentially harmful to the organ and body.

Some of the cytokines include tumor necrosis factor (TNF) and the interleukins. TNF was obviously first discovered in patients with tumors, but interestingly, now has been shown to have important prognostic importance in heart failure patients. Most interesting to me is how an understanding of these cytokines and how they are responsible for many of the symptoms of heart failure (fatigue, cachexia—muscle wasting) is leading to a better way to battle heart failure, whereas trials with drugs that block TNF have not been very encouraging so far. Stay tuned to this area of development in heart failure research. On occasion, your doctor may measure these blood levels as well.

Biopsy of the Heart Muscle

We use a heart muscle biopsy (endomyocardial biopsy) when we suspect *myocarditis* (inflammation of the heart muscle), or when we need more direct evidence about the condition or status of the heart muscle than indirect testing offers. Though some physicians don't do biopsies, because they believe the risk outweighs the reward or feel the yield is low, I've found that biopsies are useful in certain situations, yielding information that would be difficult to find without direct access to the heart muscle. In a number of instances, I've found conditions that other tests failed to reveal—sarcoid of the heart, for instance, which is a special kind of inflammation in the heart, and one for which specific treatment is available that can markedly improve the patient's condition. The stated risk for a biopsy is 0.1 percent, a risk I feel is even lower when the biopsy is performed by someone skilled in this procedure. Even more important, I believe the biopsy is one of the rare opportunities to actually see the structure of the heart and give me important information as to the degree of damage it has sustained. As I have mentioned, because of the enormous reserve the heart has, it can be quite damaged, yet the individual may actually feel fine.

In the past, the main reason people did a heart biopsy was to look for abnormal cells or inflammation in the heart muscle. Nowadays, when I look at the biopsy specimen, I do look for the abnormal cells and inflammation, but also look at the tiny blood vessels in the heart as well as how much scarring is already in the biopsy sample pieces. Often, to me, this is one of the best ways to determine the degree to which the heart is damaged, as well as how much reserve it has left.

I recall a young woman who presented with heart failure. We did a biopsy to find out if myocarditis was the cause of her problem. We found no myocarditis, but I was quite concerned, because although she seemingly recovered and was back to working hard at caring for her family of four children, I saw so much scarring in the muscle biopsy that I felt she would soon deteriorate and need a heart transplant. This did happen over the next several months, and I believe that knowing what the biopsy showed helped me to be alert to the possibility of her rapid deterioration.

Other Medical Tools

The *electrocardiogram* and chest X ray are well-known medical tools that provide a variety of useful information for heart failure patients. Electrocardiograms may reveal whether someone has had a heart attack, and can detect irregular heartbeats (either causing or being caused by heart failure), congenital defects, problems with the lining of the heart, and other data. A chest X ray helps determine the heart size, the degree of congestion, the presence of pneumonia or blood clots in the lungs, and the *cardiothoracic ratio,* that is, the amount of the chest cavity in its transverse diameter filled by the heart. The normal ratio is less than 50 percent. A heart that fills a greater proportion of the chest cavity signifies an advanced stage of heart failure. Often, a person has heard that they have an enlarged heart and may think that this means a heart that is stronger than normal, since, for instance, an "enlarged" arm muscle would probably be a stronger one. Generally, however, an enlarged heart muscle is overstressed or damaged and usually works less efficiently than a normal heart muscle. Any disease that causes heart failure may also cause an enlarged heart and, in fact, many doctors use the term as a euphemism for heart failure. Occasionally, an enlarged heart can mean a heart that is thicker than normal due to high blood pressure, and, again, this is not necessarily a more efficient heart muscle. Sometimes, a well-trained athlete may have an enlarged heart that functions normally, or even supernormally, but this is the exception to the rule.

Rather than just recording a patient's heartbeat for a few minutes in the office, physicians can use a continuous recording of heartbeats, or the twenty-four-hour Holter, to spot abnormal pauses or extra heartbeats. In recent years, cardiologists have learned that some people may even develop a form of heart failure because they have a higher than normal number of heartbeats. In some instances, when medicine reduces the heartbeat rate to a normal level, the heart failure is ameliorated or may even disappear.

Most of the diagnostic tools that we use today have been pretty standard for years. However, I'd like to mention a diagnostic tool that actually has been around since the 1960s but only now has emerged as an extremely useful tool. This is called thoracic bioimpedence. To my mind, the company that has created the best device and who has made this a reliable device is called Cardiodynamics and the device is called the BioZ.

The BioZ type device was originally designed by the NASA program to monitor the circulatory function of the astronauts without placing catheters inside of them. Using only four skin electrodes, the BioZ rapidly gives your doctors and nurses information about your heart function, how much work your heart is doing, and how much fluid you might be retaining. Many studies have shown that the results obtained with the BioZ device are every bit as accurate as those obtained with a Swan-Ganz catheter (a tube that is invasively placed inside the heart). We have written about how often the BioZ helps us avoid the need and risk to place the Swan catheter.

On a daily basis, my nurses and I use the BioZ in many situations, including intensive care units, emergency rooms, the heart failure center, and in the office. With this device we can more carefully adjust medications and make decisions about using water pills, as well as determining whether someone's increased shortness of breath is due to heart failure or to another problem. This device has been so totally helpful and changed my practice over the last few years that if you asked me if you could take away from me my stethoscope or my BioZ, I would have to admit that I'd let the stethoscope go before the BioZ—now that's saying something! Increasingly more doctors and hospitals are purchasing the BioZ and will have it available for use.

Other Markers

There are many other important markers at which your doctors and nurses may look. For example, the routine blood test measurement of sodium, or the amount of salt in the blood, may be an important indicator of how sick you are, how bad your heart failure is, and even how to better treat you. Again, blood tests that tell your doctor and nurses how well the kidneys and liver are working as organs also tell them a great deal about your condition and what steps they should follow.

Pieces of a Puzzle

There are other diagnostic tests, but I've covered the major ones. As a rule of thumb, the more tests a doctor does, the greater his or her ability to provide patients with an accurate diagnosis and effective treatment. This does not mean the more tests the better. It simply means that when doctors base their conclusions on only one test, they run the risk of jumping to erroneous conclusions. For instance, doctors who receive test results showing a low ejection fraction may tell their patients that they don't have long to live. The problem, of course, is that their one measurement may be inaccurate, or they have incorrectly diagnosed the cause of the low ejection fraction (the true cause may be treatable), or their patients may still be able to use their heart function well, meaning that their exercise capacity may be terrific.

Although multiple tests can help confirm one another, they can also create a new problem: conflicting messages. For instance, an ejection fraction may be nearly normal but the stress hormone level may be alarmingly high. It's not uncommon for conflicting results to exist, and doctors can often resolve these conflicts based on other input. They can also use additional information to confirm a suspected problem or to adjust treatment for increased efficacy.

PATIENT HISTORY

Questions to Determine the Presence of Heart Failure

In addition to our high-tech tests and equipment, and despite the fact that the heart is not the most accessible of organs, doctors can gather a startling amount of valuable data by examining and talking to patients. "How do you feel?" is one of the first and most important questions a doctor can ask you. Your answer can go a long way toward deciding what test might be needed or resolving conflicting tests and determining the most effective treatment. Therefore, never hide the truth about how you feel. Many times, patients put up a tough front and insist they haven't been feeling ill when they really have been. Or they overdramatize problems because they possess other agendas—they want to get out of work or garner sympathy. The patient history is crucial for heart failure patients; it contains subtle clues as well as obvious facts that clarify or confirm test results. The paragraphs that follow include some of the questions your doctor may specifically ask about your symptoms, as well as the rationale behind the question.

Do You Have Chest Pain or Pressure?   Your doctor may ask you if you feel pain or pressure in your chest, as well as in your neck, back, or throat. This symptom may indicate problems with the coronary arteries, but it can also occur with some types of heart valve problems, as in *hypertrophic cardiomyopathy* (a condition in which the heart muscle becomes too thick), or even with thickening of the heart due to high blood pressure. If you do have this symptom, the doctor will ask further about where the pain or pressure is and will want to know what brings it on, what makes it better, if it moves around, and how long it lasts.

Do You Have Shortness of Breath?   Your doctor may ask if you have shortness of breath, how long this has been noticed, what brings it on, what makes it better, and whether there are other symptoms that go along with it, such as chest pain or sweatiness. Commonly, patients allow this symptom to progress over weeks to months to years and seek medical attention only when there is a marked limitation (for example, unable to go out of the house without getting short of breath).

In addition to shortness of breath as you move about (we call this *exertional dyspnea*), there may be shortness of breath when you lie down on your back *(orthopnea)* or shortness of breath that occurs in the middle of the night that awakens you with a feeling of suffocation or coughing *(paroxysmal nocturnal dyspnea)*. Both of the latter result from the extra fluid that accumulates within your body and that gets back into the bloodstream when you lie down and take the force of gravity off your legs. This extra volume of blood puts an extra load on the heart, and the weakened heart forces the extra blood up into the lungs; the extra blood there causes poor oxygenation in the lungs, and the person becomes short of breath. Usually, the seated position helps, as does a walk around the room or a trip to the bathroom. Also, people who experience this symptom may place extra pillows under their head, so don't be surprised if the doctor asks about how many pillows you use at night. Getting rid of extra urine at night *(nocturia)* is also related to the nighttime return of fluid to the heart and then the kidneys, so you will be asked about this as well.

Are You Having Problems Sleeping? A sleeping problem may be related to lung congestion or to frequent nighttime urination. However, it often is related more to frequent naps or dozing off and less physical activity during the day, which means that there is less need for nighttime sleep. We also think a great many of our patients have difficulty sleeping because of concern—or even some depression—over their medical condition. It is common to see one or more of these factors preventing a normal sleep pattern. Often, when the heart failure improves and a person can get a single good night's sleep, his or her whole perspective and outlook on life improves as well.

Another important area about your sleep that your doctor should also ask about (or you mention) is what we call disordered sleep. We are becoming much more aware that disordered sleep occurs in about 40 percent of patients who have heart failure. In addition, it seems that this abnormal sleep pattern can help promote abnormalities that can actually cause or worsen heart failure (such as high blood pressure) or contribute directly to the progression of heart failure.

So what exactly is disordered sleep? It is a combination of sleep abnormalities that a patient (because they are sleeping) may not even be aware of. Basically, when a person sleeps the muscles in the throat tend to relax and in some people they can collapse so that the air cannot flow freely. This is referred to as obstructive sleep apnea. In this condition the individual often stops breathing for brief periods (apnea or hypopneas) and the oxygen levels in the blood can fall dramatically. Another form, called nonobstructive sleep apnea, seems to be a problem where the throat stays open but the brain temporarily slows down the breathing, with the same results. In my experience, both forms tend to occur in the same patient and both are common in patients with heart failure.

Aside from having heart failure, several features might make a person more likely to have disordered sleep, including obesity, fluid in the belly, or even having a short thick neck. Nevertheless, several quick questions can usually focus on whether someone might have this problem. The first question goes to the patient's partner or spouse. The question is "Does the patient snore?" Usually, if disordered sleep is present they will readily respond that they do, and that it is quite loud and in fact the breathing does sometimes stop. One of my patient's wives told me the first time they came to see me that she was so tired because she stayed awake every night for the last eight years to watch her husband breathe at night to make sure he was not going to stop breathing!

The other questions are whether upon awakening the person feels rested and whether they have daytime drowsiness. If any of these questions are positive it is worth considering the possibility of disordered sleep. Obviously, lots of these symptoms are the same ones related to the heart failure, such as tiredness and daytime naps. I usually work to get the heart failure in good shape and then go back and investigate the possibility of disordered sleep.

If there is a concern about disordered sleep, then a patient can be referred to a sleep laboratory, which is a place where a person actually sleeps for a night, wired up to monitors for oxygen, heart rate, chest movement, snoring, and so on. Then the doctors can accurately tell whether there is a problem with the breathing. If the test is positive several solutions are available, including the use of a CPAP (continuous positive airway pressure) mask. These masks, which fit only over the nose, deliver a steady stream of air that is sufficient to keep the airway open. They also work in the nonobstructed forms. Often a second sleep study is required to titrate the air pressure. All this seems cumbersome, but it can really improve how many people feel and improve their heart failure. More advances are being made every day. Some trials are beginning to use simpler home monitors to do a screening test for sleep apnea in patients at high risk, such as those with heart failure (Nexan). I believe this is important adjunctive therapy.

Are You More Fatigued Lately?   Fatigue is simply one of the many manifestations that the heart is not doing its job as a pump of blood. The muscles and even the brain may not get enough blood or enough oxygen, which is the fuel the body operates on, and this will result in fatigue. People commonly attribute fatigue to being out of shape or getting older, since it can sneak up on a person slowly over the years. Fatigue after even minimal activity can cause a person to doze off easily or catnap frequently during the day. This can lead to poor sleep at night and can start a vicious cycle of confusion of days and nights (day-night reversal).

Have You Gained or Lost Weight Recently?   With heart failure, there is usually a decline in the appetite, and weight loss may occur. More commonly, however, there is accumulation of fluid in the body owing to the poor heart function, and the person notices weight gain despite eating almost nothing. Fluid accumulation may be noticed in the hands (rings are tighter) or in the feet (the person may switch to wearing looser shoes or tennis shoes), or it may simply be that clothes (skirts, dresses, pants) that used to fit are now tight. Obviously, many conditions can cause weight loss or gain, but, surprisingly, this may be the first thing a person or a family member notices. I started treating an elderly woman recently because her daughter, who provided all her meals and therefore knew how little she really was eating, noticed that none of her clothes fit anymore. Since the elderly woman was relatively inactive, shortness of breath was really not one of her initial complaints.

Have You Noticed Changes in Your Appetite?   Most commonly, people with advanced heart failure notice a loss of appetite. They describe a bloated feeling or a feeling of filling up fast after eating very little (we call this *early satiety*). People who would consistently take second or third helpings can now barely finish half the food on their plate. The reasons for this are many but include more inactivity; the high energy costs of digesting food, which a person with a weakened pump can't afford; swelling of the intestine, from the extra retained body fluid or blood; and swelling of the liver, for the same reason, which leads to the liver enlarging and pressing on the stomach, so that the stomach's capacity is reduced.

People with these problems should be told to eat smaller, more frequent meals and foods that are easier to digest. Once the initial fluid overload is reduced with proper treatment, this problem often disappears rapidly for many people.

Do Your Legs Ever Swell?   Swelling of the legs is a finding that can represent a variety of causes and does not always reflect a form of heart failure. When it is related to the heart, it can start out as just a little tightness at the ankles at the end of the day, after standing for most of the day. Later, it progresses to a swelling that remains even in the morning and then to swelling that encompasses the entire body, including a marked swelling of the belly (even the genitalia may become swollen when this condition is severe).

Questions Following a Diagnosis of Heart Failure

Now I will review some of the more important questions doctors ask once a diagnosis of heart failure has been made and the relevance of the answers to diagnosis and treatment.

How Did Your Heart Failure Begin and at What Age? What Were the First Symptoms, and How Did They Evolve?   To more precisely characterize a patient's heart failure, the doctor will want to know what the patient's first symptoms were, when they began, and how they developed. The following are some typical responses to this line of inquiry and what they mean to the doctor: A sixty-year-old man notes that he has had high blood pressure since he was forty, began feeling "sluggish" in his fifties, and had his first episode of heart failure at fifty-eight. He says, "My internist checked my heart and said it was fine." On the basis of this history, I would suspect that this man has hypertensive heart disease, that he started out with a diastolic abnormality, and that he may now have systolic and diastolic abnormalities.

Another man responds that he had his first heart attack at forty, another one when he was fifty-two, and a third at fifty-five. He complains of swollen legs and feeling winded and tired since the third attack. It's likely this man is suffering from ischemic heart disease; that is, his heart failure is a result of multiple injuries to the heart muscle due to blocked coronary arteries.

A woman complains that her episodes seem to have "come out of the blue." She says she feels fine during the daytime hours but at around 11:00 P.M., after being asleep for about an hour, she finds herself gasping for breath; her husband has had to call the paramedics. This woman is probably suffering from *flash pulmonary edema,* which means the sudden backup of blood from the heart into the lungs, which causes severe lung congestion. This could be a result of diastolic dysfunction or perhaps coronary disease, hypertension, or both.

These brief case histories are simply examples to show you how the symptoms you tell your doctor really are the guideposts he or she will use for determining further testing and treatment. Besides describing the symptoms, you should communicate to your physician when they began, how long they've been going on, and whether they appeared suddenly or gradually. When you tell your doctor about your symptoms, you may be doing nothing more than confirming what he or she already suspects. But you may also be giving your doctor that nugget of information that allows him or her to make the right decision about your treatment and to give you an indication of how sick (or how relatively healthy) you are.

What Other Medical Problems Have You Had in the Past?   Heart failure specialists are alert to diseases, symptoms, and medications that may have caused or exacerbated a patient's current condition, or that may be valuable clues for diagnosis and prognosis. Some of the red flags are diabetes, thyroid condition, viral illnesses, coronary disease and related factors (smoking, high blood pressure, high cholesterol), drug and alcohol abuse (or even just use), and kidney disease. For instance, the heart failure patient who reports that she had a viral illness preceding her symptoms of heart failure may be the victim of myocarditis (heart muscle inflammation). Sometimes, the link between a previous medical problem and heart failure may be more subtle. A middle-aged woman recently came to my office after experiencing her first heart failure episode. After taking her medical history, the cause of her condition was still a mystery to me until she mentioned that she had had Hodgkin's disease almost thirty years before. It turns out that she had received relatively high doses of radiation and that the radiation had damaged her heart muscle and coronary arteries. Suspecting that she might have radiation heart disease, I ordered specific tests and was able to help her considerably.

Has Anyone Else in Your Family Experienced Heart Failure? Most people realize that coronary heart disease runs in families, but until recently, the same link wasn't established for forms of heart failure. Although there is some debate over this issue, my experience has been that dilated cardiomyopathy often runs in families.

What Do You Do for a Living, and How Do You Feel at Work? Although it might not appear to be relevant at first blush, occupations can reveal a great deal about a heart failure patient's condition. When patients start talking about specific activities in the workplace (from walking to the office to putting products on shelves to loading trucks to running to catch the train), they frequently remember to relate a physical problem they've been experiencing there: "Doctor, I've noticed recently that whenever I start erasing the blackboard, I feel dizzy and winded." Any upper extremity activity can trigger heart-related pain or shortness of breath, and people generally clearly remember when such a symptom first began at work, thus giving doctors a time line to chart the onset of the disease. Of course, patients may first become aware of such a symptom when it relates to some physical activity in the home as well. I've had patients relate their symptoms to such things as washing dishes, washing their hair, and performing housework. This type of information also gives doctors a benchmark against which they can measure how patients fare after treatment. The doctor will want to know if the patient still feels winded when erasing the blackboard (or loading the truck or stocking the shelves, and so on), or if the feeling is gone or lessened.

The environment in which a patient works can also contribute to a diagnosis. Certain airborne chemicals or dusts can contribute to heart failure problems. In addition, people who work in cold environments (very cold rooms or outside in winter) experience more heart failure symptoms than people in warm environments. This is because cold causes blood vessels to constrict, which increases the heart's workload. I've seen patients for whom a change in environment results in a near-miraculous improvement in how they feel.

PHYSICAL EXAM

Heart failure often manifests itself in surprisingly visible, audible, and tactile ways. The following paragraphs describe some of the signs doctors look for when examining heart failure patients.

High Blood Pressure

Hypertension over a period of years does more than contribute to coronary disease; it also weakens the heart. Unfortunately, many heart failure patients never realize they have high blood pressure. Part of the problem is the prevalent attitude in the medical community that moderately high blood pressure is acceptable, particularly in the elderly. The common notion that your blood pressure should be 100 plus your age is an absolute myth and one that should be destroyed. Years of moderate hypertension can lead to heart failure in people in their forties and fifties, and is a common cause of heart failure in people over sixty-five. Allthough we generally say that blood pressure should not exceed 140/90, this does not mean that our goal should be 139/89. Indeed, in the latest authoritative report on high blood pressure treatment (JNC 6) the 140/90 is called high normal and for some patients with certain risk factors such as diabetes and protein in the urine the normal ranges are now set much lower. In many countries where salt is not a major dietary substance, normal blood pressure is 90/60 for life. Normally, the top number (systolic blood pressure) should be between 90 and 120, and the bottom number (diastolic blood pressure) between 60 and 80. Ask your doctor for more specific details.

If I had to point to one single item that I thought contributes more to heart failure than any other it would be high blood pressure and in fact adequate control of high blood pressure may be the single most important step you can take regarding your health.

Rapid Resting Heart Rate

When the body senses heart failure, the heart responds by beating faster. Resting *tachycardia,* or fast heartbeat of 90 or 100, especially if it stays at that high level for a period of time, signals a serious problem. At rest, the heart rate normally slows. The actual rate depends on age, the status of the heart, and the individual's overall level of conditioning. Generally, a resting heart should beat between fifty to seventy beats per minute. You can check your heart rate by feeling the pulse in your neck or wrist, or by listening to the heart with a stethoscope. An electrocardiogram will also measure heart rate.

Unusual Skin Color and Abnormalities

Cyanotic, or blue skin suggests a form of heart failure that can be due to a congenital defect; it also suggests a lung problem that can ultimately cause a special kind of heart failure known as right-sided heart failure, or *cor pulmonale*. A fingertip or fingernail examination (checking for color, shape, or appearance changes) can reveal some circulatory causes, whereas some skin lesions can indicate an esoteric form of heart failure, such as that related to scleroderma or lupus erythematosus.

Congested Lungs

Lung congestion may mean that the heart is weak and that blood has backed into the lungs. Blood normally flows from the right side of the heart, through the lungs, into the left side of the heart. If the left side of the heart becomes weakened, however, blood flow may reverse in part and back up, or congest, the lungs. When there is too much pressure backup, more fluid leaks into the lung tissue and may cause a cough, shortness of breath, or even a feeling of suffocation. In these situations, doctors call what they hear when listening to the lungs with a stethoscope *rales* or *crackles*.

"Raised" Neck Veins

Neck veins are to the heart what a dipstick is to a car. They help monitor how much fluid is inside the circulation. If there's too much blood and pressure builds up on the right side of the heart, the neck veins become swollen or engorged. We primarily look at the internal jugular vein, but we can look at other veins of the body to give us some clues to the "volume status" of the person. This tells us how much extra blood or fluid is within the circulation.

Abnormal Heart Sounds

Listening to the heart through a stethoscope placed on various areas of the chest can reveal a murmur, which means abnormal blood flow; extra sounds, which may indicate a weakness; or "rubs," which reflect extra fluid accumulating around the heart.

Swelling of Various Body Parts

Swelling may be seen in the abdomen, in the back *(presacral edema)*, in the arms, legs, or feet, or even in the genitalia. Swelling in the liver can be palpated.

TABLE 3.1 Heart Failure Type, Causes, and Diagnostic Tests

Heart failure type	Cause	Diagnostic test
Ischemic cardiomyopathy	One or more heart attacks	Angiogram (heart catheterization); stress echocardiogram
Hypertensive cardiomyopathy	High blood pressure	Blood and urine tests; echocardiogram
Dilated cardiomyopathy (idiopathic cardiomyopathy)	Unknown	Possibly endomyocardial biopsy; echocardiogram; angiogram
Valvular cardiomyopathy	Either congential or acquired valve damage	Echocardiogram; cardiac catheterization
Cor pulmonale	Emphysema or other causes of lung tissue damage	Echocardiogram; Swan–Ganz catheter measurements
Hypertrophic cardiomyopathy	Genetic or result of spontaneous development	Echocardiogram

Usually, this swelling, which is caused by the retention of excess fluid and salt, affects the entire body, but it may be best detected in one specific area or another. For example, a person with leg swelling usually already has liver swelling, and so on, but he or she may not be aware of this liver swelling until the leg swelling is appreciable.

THE MORE YOU KNOW, THE BETTER OFF YOU'LL BE

Knowledge is power. These tests, exams, and questions have a cumulative value for both patient and physician. The information gleaned from this process provides patients with a much better understanding of the condition. I've found that patients need that understanding.

They have an innate desire to know the cause of their heart failure, what their prospects are, how advanced the disease is, what can be done, what the alternatives are, what they should expect, and what their obligations and duties are. Table 3.1 summarizes the types of heart failure, their causes, and the tests used to diagnose them.

From a treatment perspective, these data are essential. Contrary to myth, heart failure is treatable and, in some cases, reversible. A battery of tests and questions may help us identify those people who are suffering from reversible forms of heart failure. Though these people are in the minority, they still comprise a significant percentage of heart failure patients. Instead of assuming their condition will get progressively worse and treating them accordingly, we can look for the sometimes subtle signs that indicate a reversible problem, for example, an inactive or too active thyroid gland.

We've gained so much knowledge and made so much progress with drug and other therapies that it would be a shame to waste those accomplishments because we've misdiagnosed heart failure patients or failed to acquire the necessary information for effective treatment. The SAVE study, a recent study of people who had heart attacks, reinforces this point. The study divided its subjects into two groups: those who received medications to prevent progressive heart enlargement and weakening, and those who did not. The study concluded that the medicated group had much less enlargement and a significantly lower rate of heart failure than the nonmedicated group. Yet in spite of this clear demonstration of the value of such medication, many heart attack survivors who never have another heart attack die prematurely from heart failure because no one has monitored their heart size or treated them for this problem.

The more we know, the easier it is to tailor treatment for a specific heart failure patient, that is, to treat our patients holistically. We can determine, for instance, if a patient is in NYHA Functional Class I, II, III, or IV (with I being the least serious). If we know someone is in Class IV, we would probably design an aggressive treatment regimen; perhaps we would consider experimental approaches and use higher doses of medication. For someone in Class I, on the other hand, we might be much more concerned about the day-to-day quality-of-life issues and might therefore try to reduce medications and diuretics to a minimum.

Finally, our ability to predict the specific cause of heart failure death can also aid in our treatment approach. On the basis of the tools discussed in this chapter, we can often determine that a given heart failure patient is most vulnerable to death from one of the following: progressive heart failure (the majority of patients die because of the progressive weakening of the heart muscle); arrhythmia (a series of irregular heartbeats); or one of a variety of more unusual causes, such as a blood clot that embolizes and enters the lungs. If, for instance, we can determine that you are most likely to be victimized by arrhythmia, we can try drugs or implant a defibrillator, a device that senses an irregular heartbeat and automatically delivers an electrical shock that restores a normal beat. Defibrillators have been found to decrease mortality rates for heart failure patients. Defibrillators are generally used when the heartbeat is too fast, in contrast to pacemakers, which prevent the heartbeat from becoming too slow.

4

How Attitude and Emotion Affect Heart Failure:
Mind-Body Relationships

SEX AND HEART FAILURE

There is no doubt in my mind whatsoever that emotions, stress, attitudes, beliefs, fears, and mental attitude affect bodily functions. Although the so-called mind-body relationship has been difficult to quantify over the years, there is currently an outpouring of elegant scientific studies showing how things that happen in the mind affect things that happen in the body. Much of this impressive science is called pyschoneuroimmunobiology. In fact, one of my most fun professional activities over the past several years has been serving on the editorial advisory board of *Alternative Therapies in Health and Medicine,* a remarkable scientific journal focused on better documenting and substantiating the role of complementary and alternative approaches to health and healing.

What this fancy word, psychoneuroimmunobiology, tells us is that thoughts and emotions are capable of creating chemical reactions that can travel in our bodies and create physical actions. Much of this science has looked, for example, at how a person's emotions affect the development of problems such as cancer or allergies with the immune system.

None of this should really seem strange to any of us—that thoughts and emotions can affect us physically. With all the science related to this field, I think it is hard to deny the existence of a mind-body relationship. Examples are all around us. If, in fact, you deny this relationship, then you probably should not be reading this book, since I believe that the knowledge and emotional strength you get from reading this kind of book can be transformed into better heart function. Many people know of Dr. Dean Ornish, a skilled cardiologist, who revolutionized our whole thinking of heart disease by showing that some forms of heart disease, blockages in the coronary arteries, are, in fact, reversible! Reversible, yes, with diet, exercise, and meditation. (Required reading for many of my patients are Dr. Ornish's books, including *Dr. Dean Ornish's Program for Reversing Heart Disease*, 1990). Ornish has written another book entitled *Love and Survival: The Scientific Basis for the Healing Power of Intimacy*. In this book Dr. Ornish highlights how the range of emotions from rage and hostility on one end to love and acceptance on the other can serve to promote or worsen cardiac disease or prevent and heal it! This, then, is not a pill or an injection, but use of the most powerful set of medicinals—our own minds and emotions. A goal, therefore, for heart failure patients, or anyone, for that matter, is to find the ways, and there are many, to harness their own powerful medicine to help them. There are so many books written about the paths to take in this direction that I cannot give you a single method that works best for everyone. But I would suggest the simple foundation, which includes the following:

1. *Owning your shadow,* which is pulling out your greatest fears, expressing them, and facing them. If, for example, after reading about heart failure, you are "scared to death" about the risk of sudden death, then set aside some time to talk about this with family and your doctor. By knowing this fear, perhaps other approaches or trials can be tried to at least put you in control of the fear and let you do something about it.

2. The other approach is simply to *know the facts.* This means that you should become one of the world's authorities on heart failure. Seriously, many of my patients know much, much more current and factual information about heart failure than many health professionals in this country. This book, and really most of what I do to help people, is to help them get their own power, to "allow" them to be proactive, take control, and *know the facts!*

Other powerful examples of mind-body interactions are how spiritual emotions and often religious participation such as prayer can affect health and healing. One of my personal heroes is Dr. Larry Dossey, a medical doctor (and executive editor of *Alternative Therapies in Health and Medicine*), who has come out of the closet on exploring the impact prayer can have on health and healing. Dossey has written several superb books exploring the scientific evidence that prayer, even prayer that is nonlocal (that is, done at a distance, without the person being prayed for having any knowledge of the prayer) can be very effective. (I suggest you read *Healing Words* or *Prayer Is Good Medicine* by Larry Dossey to find out more about these concepts and explore this very important topic.)

Other forms of mind-body relationships are nonspiritual. Examples abound and are quite common in everyday life. For example, who has not heard of someone who has a headache or belly pain or gas related to emotional stress or pressure in his or her life? Women who have used the Lamaze method of childbirth have practiced mind-body medicine; in this method, by concentrating on a "focal spot" or something of pleasure, or something relaxing, they can markedly diminish the sensations of pain in their bodies. Or doesn't hearing an old, favorite song (music therapy) or smelling a favorite smell (aromatherapy) cause a better mood and improvement in your daily functioning?

One of the most well-studied and important effects in clinical medicine may well be the "placebo effect." Over a wide range of conditions and diseases, using well-controlled "double-blind" (where neither the patient nor the doctor knows which pill is the placebo) studies, there is in almost every situation between a 20 and 40 percent placebo effect, that is, that patients respond as if they had received a real or active medicine rather than an inert sugar pill. Even in heart failure, there is a well-known placebo effect in trials. This effect evades clarification, but for me is still another classic example of how the mind can talk to and even direct bodily function.

Therefore, it seems important to face the fact that attitude and understanding by heart failure patients can have a significant effect on how they function, live with their disease, and potentially even affect their outcome.

When patients hear the term *heart failure,* they are frequently devastated. The word *failure* has an ominous ring, and many people automatically assume, "This is it; there's nothing left to be done." They may even sink into a deep depression from which they never extricate themselves. There have been studies that demonstrate a link between the mood and physical condition of patients with various diseases, and empirical evidence leads me to believe that such a connection certainly exists for heart failure patients. Time after time, I've seen optimistic, positive-minded patients feel better and live longer than pessimistic, negative-minded ones. I'm not sure why this is so. Perhaps the correlation is similar to that between stress and heart attacks: Studies have demonstrated clearly that stress is a risk factor for heart disease. Or it might be that the heart is an organ exquisitely attuned to our emotions, that the folklore about people getting "heartsick" because of a lost love has more truth to it than we think.

Whatever the reason, a positive mental attitude is therapeutic. In this chapter, I'd like to explain why this is so and how patients, physicians, family, therapists, and support groups can combine their efforts to foster this attitude.

NEGATIVE ATTITUDES

Fear, anger, denial, and depression are some of the understandable reactions to a heart failure diagnosis. Fear of the unknown is a natural response. Patients are afraid of the myriad tests and treatments they face; of the reactions of friends, family, and employers; and of their own mortality. We commonly see anger in dilated cardiomyopathy patients. They've avoided bad habits such as smoking and a high-cholesterol diet, and have never had high blood pressure, yet their hearts are failing; the injustice causes them to strike out. Another possible response to the diagnosis is denial. Patients who use denial insist that they're fine and give their doctor misleading signals about their condition. They insist to others, and perhaps even to themselves, that they can "tough it out." Finally, there's depression, probably the most common emotional response to a diagnosis of heart failure, and the most destructive. Depressed patients convince themselves there is no hope, and such a conviction can become a self-fulfilling prophecy.

In many ways, these responses mirror the traditional grieving process. Acceptance of their condition doesn't come for many patients until they've worked through these and other emotions. Sometimes, there's a false acceptance initially, usually by patients who have been suffering for years and who now feel better as a result of treatment. A diuretic can quickly and effectively relieve excess fluid, bringing comfort to patients, but it may not improve the patient's heart function. Because they feel so much better, these patients may then indulge in a high-salt diet or discard their medicine; they assume that they have improved sufficiently to cheat on their regimen and that their doctor can bail them out again if necessary. When their symptoms grow worse, the seriousness of their situation hits them for the first time.

I've found that heart attack survivors are often especially bitter when they learn they have heart failure. They may have assumed they were well after a successful coronary bypass and only later learn that the trauma of the heart attack has weakened the heart muscle to the point that it's failing.

Depression (to be discussed), anger, and other negative emotions harm treatment in two ways. First, patients stop doing what they should be doing or resume habits they should have given up. They don't take their medicine (or take it only sporadically); they ignore salt, fluid, and other dietary restrictions; they miss appointments with their doctors or fail to provide them with accurate information about their symptoms; they fail to get proper exercise and are no longer active and involved; and they continue bad habits such as smoking or drinking.

The second problem is that when patients give up in their minds, they also frequently give up in their bodies. It's as if they're sending a signal from their heads to their hearts that it's not worth the effort. This mental surrender, combined with the practical problems caused by not following a prescribed medical regimen, can shorten life and destroy quality of life.

To avoid this situation or remedy it, patients, physicians, nurses, and family must understand how and why heart failure patients often become so pessimistic and depressed. Many times, certain factors make a bad situation worse.

COMMON CATALYSTS

Sleep deprivation can make healthy people moody and irritable; the effect on people with heart failure can be even more severe. Heart failure patients often have trouble sleeping at night for the following reasons: Some experience fluid backing up in their lungs and therefore have difficulty breathing; those taking diuretics wake up frequently at night to go to the bathroom; and some have an often unarticulated fear that if they go to sleep, they won't wake up.

Certain drugs that patients take can sometimes exacerbate negative emotions. Possible side effects of heart-related drugs include mood swings, confusion (especially in elderly people), altered taste sensations, and problems with balance and gait. A drug such as an ACE (angiotensin-converting enzyme) inhibitor can create a nagging, chronic cough. Diuretics often cause the mouth to be dry and make people feel they must limit their activities because of frequent trips to the bathroom. Perhaps the most depressed people are those with the greatest change in functional capacity, namely, vigorous men and women who worked and played hard, and who have been told (or have decided on their own) to quit work and "take it easy." For many men, especially, the inability to work and the corresponding economic hardship are crushing blows. One of my patients is an insurance salesman in his early fifties with kids to put through college. Because of his heart failure, he lost his job (it requires a great deal of energy to make sales calls, and his primary symptom is fatigue). Ironically, he also lost his insurance coverage, which adds to the economic pressure he is experiencing.

Idle time often allows patients to dwell on their conditions and symptoms. We see patients who never complained about anything in their lives suddenly become filled with self-pity. Feeling a loss of independence is a major problem as well. Often, this is unwittingly fostered by well-meaning spouses, doctors, and nurses who try too hard to reinforce restrictions on the patient's diet and activity. Recently, I saw a man whose heart failure was getting worse. I could not put my finger on any particular cause for this deterioration. I found out from his wife that he had stopped exercising. Why? I asked him, and he said it was because he had no time. Well, he was retired, and time really wasn't the issue, so I probed further. He said he spent all his time working on his insurance claims and figuring out how to pay for "all the damn medicines." Again, I sensed this was not the "real" issue and so probed again. It turned out that this man had a dear friend who had passed away, and this sent my patient into a deep despair. As he began to focus on his illness and his health, he allowed this, rather than to help him, to slow him down; he stopped exercising and eventually it impacted how he did feel. We talked about these issues and I was able to get him to realize that the power was his, which made his heart failure symptoms better.

Finally, the loss of sexual function can radically alter patients' moods. As I ask, I find that poor sexual functioning is a major or minor concern for almost all my patients. *This is a problem!* The reason this is a problem is that when sexual function is impaired, it affects emotions, intimacy, and support—the precise things my patients need in their lives. As many of my patients know, I feel this is important, since I view sexual activity, at least in part, as a way of getting controlled physical activity. Yes, sex is exercise, and it can be done by virtually all patients using some common sense.

I want to examine some of the reasons patients often complain about sexual dysfunction. Poor blood flow to sexual organs and certain medications can result in impotence or a decrease in pleasure. More often than not, though, this condition is psychological rather than physiological. It usually revolves around patients' fears that sexual activity may lead to further damage to their heart or do them some harm. This starts the cascade of negative emotions among partners, and before long, many other aspects of a couple's life besides the aspects of the physical illness are suffering. Nonetheless, the damage has been done, and both men and women suffer from moodiness because of this loss. I must mention, however, that in the last few years, working with a skilled urologist, Dr. John Mulhall, who is an expert on sexual dysfunction, I have learned much more about the impact drugs can have on sexual dysfunction and much more about simple and straightforward methods available to treat these problems. I cannot tell you how many of my patients feel that getting some improvement in their sexual lives has made them feel better with their heart failure. In fact, I can think of several men and women who would say that addressing the sexual aspects of their lives helped them refocus on so many other areas and truly change their lives from a focus on illness to a focus on health. The bottom line here is that if your doctor does not question you on any issues related to sexual function, you should take the bull by the horns and bring it up in the question-and-answer portion of your visit!

Finally, I should add a word about Viagra, which is about the biggest news item lately. This drug essentially causes blood vessels to dilate or enlarge, letting more blood flow into an organ. In the case of Viagra, this effect occurs predominantly in the penis and hence improves male erection and sexual function. Unfortunately, Viagra can greatly increase the effect of nitroglycerin so that in patients taking both drugs, there can be a sudden and dangerous drop in blood pressure. A similar drop in blood pressure can occur with heart failure patients who are on other forms of blood pressure–lowering drugs.

So, although Viagra seems so popular, patients with heart failure must be very careful about combining this medicine with others they are on. Since there are so many ways to battle sexual dysfunction, be sure to discuss this matter openly with your doctor.

GETTING OFF TO A POSITIVE START

Fortunately, we've developed a number of successful tactics to combat some of the problems related to poor mental attitude, worry, depression, anxiety, and so on. Again, I am not a psychiatrist or psychologist. These are just things that have worked for my patients. Let's examine what these tactics are and how you and your doctors and nurses can use them.

What doctors tell heart failure patients during their initial meeting has a tremendous influence on patients' attitudes. It's easy for people to jump to conclusions and to think their conditions are far worse than they really are. Because patients are usually quite upset, they can easily misinterpret or fail to understand what their doctors tell them. I've also found that some physicians inadvertently emphasize the negative over the positive, telling patients only what's wrong with them.

Individuals with heart failure don't improve unless they see the possibility for improvement. They won't take their medicine and will ignore fluid and salt restrictions if they think they have only a few months of low-quality life left. That's why, if there's a chance for improvement—and there usually is—patients should be aware of it. In almost every case, I'm able to tell a patient during the first meeting, "I think there's something I can do for you."

I also ask a very simple question: "If I could help you do something you either can't do now or are worried you won't be able to do, what would it be?" The responses run the gamut—from playing golf to going back to work to attending a grandchild's wedding. Setting goals is crucial. They give patients reasons for living and nonmedical barometers to measure how they're doing. Many times, when people surprise themselves and achieve that first goal, they're motivated to reach the next one. If Mary finds that she is able to walk around the block, she'll be willing to work toward the goal of walking to the store by herself. Or if a person can gradually go back to work part time, there is hope that he or she will eventually go back full time or realize that part-time work is suitable and acceptable. Even a brief visit to relatives or a trip to a shopping mall gives the patient hope that he or she is not permanently housebound.

When I've determined the specific condition of a heart failure patient and clearly communicated it to him or her, I then create short-, medium-, and long-range treatment plans and explain each one. This takes the mystery out of treatment and transforms a scary and uncertain future into something more structured and understandable. At the same time, I outline the treatment options associated with each plan. Too often, patients give up hope when treatment option number one doesn't work; they assume such an option was their best and last hope. They don't realize that there are usually many other options with equal chances for success.

SIMPLE TREATMENT ADJUSTMENTS

Treatment plans shouldn't be set in stone. Even if a change in treatment won't significantly improve a patient's condition directly, it may do so indirectly; when patients feel better, they're more optimistic about life, and that optimism motivates them to do everything possible to get better.

Of course, no medically related change should be made without carefully evaluating a patient's condition. Treatment plans for some people must maintain a delicate balance; for them, even the slightest variation can have serious repercussions. For most patients, relatively minor changes do little harm and can do much good. I've found that the following adjustments can make a world of difference in the emotional well-being of heart failure patients.

Vary the Times for Taking Diuretics

Many patients become sleep deprived because diuretics cause them to wake up a number of times at night to go to the bathroom. Others are embarrassed at work, afraid to go to work, or even skip doses because of worries about incontinence. Taking diuretics at more convenient times can eliminate or lessen these problems. In some cases, the doses can be decreased. I've also found that, for certain people, diuretics work better in the afternoon than in the morning. If the morning diuretic is causing problems at work, the patient may be better off taking it only in the afternoon.

Ease Up on Dietary Restrictions

Restrictions must make sense. When the limits doctors place on patients regarding eating and drinking are too numerous or too strict, they can negatively and significantly alter their moods. One of my patients came into my office a few weeks after he'd been limiting his salt intake to under two grams daily and said, "I've been feeling much better, but you've made my life miserable." It turned out that he loved ketchup almost as much as life itself, and he was really upset about not being able to put it on his food. Allowing him to have a little ketchup now and then significantly improved his outlook. Many times, I've found that simply telling patients not to add any salt to their food from a saltshaker reduces their salt intake to an acceptable level. For others, there are one or two key dishes that need to be avoided (see Chapter 11). I would say that most family disagreements regarding treatment for heart failure center around dietary restrictions.

Vary Dosages and Brands of Drugs

Even minor variations in the dosage or brand of drug used can produce a change that helps the patient begin to succeed. For example, if a patient gets a cough with one of the ACE inhibitor drugs, then he or she should get the cough with all the various brands of these drugs. However, I frequently switch brands, trying three or even more, and surprisingly, many people end up on the needed drug without a cough! We should also not overlook the placebo effect. A study recently at Ohio State University proved that the placebo effect, or the belief by patients that a pill may help, actually did improve heart function in heart failure patients.

Maintain Rather Than Limit Activities

If you take away a person's job, hobbies, exercise routine, and family and social life, what does he or she have left? Every physician should determine what activity is important to a patient and do everything possible to help him or her continue that activity. A significant percentage of heart failure patients are remarkably active. Some recent studies have demonstrated that progressive exercise therapy can actually improve cardiac function, and, in fact, is one of the important treatments for this condition (see Chapter 10). In my experience and that of my colleagues, active, participating patients do much better than passive, disinterested ones.

SUPPORT GROUPS AND THERAPY

Given the millions of people diagnosed with heart failure, you would think that there would be a correspondingly large number of support groups for those patients and their families. Unfortunately, that's not the case. Relatively few groups exist (see Appendix II), and those that do are highly specialized. Young Hearts, for instance, is a group originating in Chicago for people under forty with heart abnormalities. Although there are heart transplant support groups, these organizations, as the name implies, exclude anyone who hasn't had or isn't waiting for a heart transplant.

Having started the first heart failure support groups in Chicago, I saw the tremendous psychological benefits they offer group members. The ideal support group serves two purposes: It brings in experts—doctors, nurses, nutritionists—to answer practical questions about heart failure, and it allows members to exchange common concerns and experiences. As a result, people no longer feel they're alone and helpless; they enjoy the camaraderie that develops and the opportunity to share their feelings with people who have a similar diagnosis, and who therefore understand in ways that others cannot. We are now part of a large NIH trial called HART that focuses on the benefits of learning ways of dealing with stress as an important aid for heart failure.

Family and friends can form another type of support group. They can help the heart failure patient look forward instead of backward, and they are able to ameliorate the bitterness and anger that mitigate against successful treatment. From a purely practical standpoint, they can help patients deal with what is often a confusing regimen of pills, doctor appointments, and dietary restrictions. By helping patients get used to a new routine (which pills to take and when, for instance), they enable them to achieve a comfort level in those crucial first few weeks.

Some patients require more help than support groups or family members can provide, or they may not have access to support groups or family. Psychological counseling is an option a patient should consider and the physician should recommend when a patient's negative state of mind is interfering with his or her treatment. Seeing a psychologist, social worker, or psychiatrist can be very helpful, especially when a patient is acutely depressed. At the same time, however, therapy can be expensive and may not be covered by insurance. In the case of the heart failure patient who is only mildly depressed, or the one who is extremely worried about money, strong support is needed from friends, family, professionals, and, occasionally, short-term drugs that help the depression without worsening the heart muscle function.

SOCIETAL ATTITUDES

Society can make heart failure patients feel like second-class citizens. A patient of mine who was in excellent shape after a transplant experienced numerous job rejections and told me she felt like an ex-con. Primarily because of worries about insurance costs, companies are wary of hiring anyone with a diagnosis of heart failure. Insurance companies hear the term *heart failure* and run the other way, even without knowing about or listening to the objective assessment or prognostic indicators. Similarly, there are relatively few support groups and rehabilitation programs tailored to heart failure patients' needs because of the false assumption that there's nothing to be done for these people. Is it any wonder that heart failure patients feel depressed?

My hope is that as more and more people are diagnosed with heart failure, organizations and institutions will change their attitudes and create supportive programs and policies. Such programs and policies can go a long way toward improving the outlook, that is, both the prospects and perspective, of heart failure patients.

Finally, I recommend a book that I first read about in an Ann Landers column. Called *Taking Charge* by Irene Pollin and Susan Golant (Times Books, 1995), it is written for people with chronic diseases and helps them to ask some of the right questions I recommend to get back the answers they need.

DEPRESSION

Quite simply, nearly 40 percent of patients who have heart failure also have depression. I am not a psychiatrist or a psychologist, but it seems clear to me that depression is rampant in our country (and as I have traveled, in many other countries as well). I do not pretend to understand all the reasons or biochemical alterations responsible for the many forms of depression, but according to the American Psychiatric Association, this disease strikes more than 17 million Americans. In fact, one in four women and one in ten men will experience depression at some point in their lives.

These are the "official" statistics, but my concern is about the millions more who suffer with a chronic disease such as heart failure and whose poor attitude, loss of motivation, poor sleep habits, noncompliant dietary habits, and medicine-taking habits are adversely affected because of depression. Moreover, who would not feel some sadness or depression if at the peak of their lives a disease called heart failure works its way into every moment of their lives, limiting their activity, restricting their diet and lifestyle, and adding bills and worries to their lives? I believe that chronic diseases such as heart failure, emphysema, diabetes, and renal failure all are risk factors for depression, and this additional "disease" should be sought actively in all of them. It is interesting that when one reads a textbook about Chinese medicine and they describe "heart-qi deficiency," which is the Chinese analogue for heart failure, the ancient Chinese doctors list depression as one of its symptoms!

Many heart failure patients, as well as their family members, suffer from depression at some point and the depression mostly goes unrecognized, untreated, and, most important, undiscussed. The problems exist on several levels. First of all, for patients to get help for depression, either they, their family members, or a doctor or nurse must recognize the depression *and* someone must act or at least mention the term to the person.

I can't tell you how many times I have simply said to a patient, "Are you depressed?" and without a moment's hesitation, hint of shame, or reluctance, the answer comes back, "Yes," or "I think so. Can you help?" I think most physicians often consider depression in a patient but are afraid to ask or put it into words, simply because they are fearful they may offend the patient. For this reason and perhaps many others, it is estimated that two-thirds of Americans who have depression never get any treatment.

Within my own practice, I frequently ask patients about depression, but I know that is not enough. There are many tools to better screen a patient for clinical depression, including the Beck Depression Scale and the Geriatric Depression Scale. These are quick and easy to use, and at least give the doctor some idea of the potential problem.

Treatment is another matter, and it is controversial. First of all, I find no risk in asking someone if he or she is depressed. With changing attitudes about depression in our country, if a person has been willing to accept help for other medical problems such as heart disease, drug or alcohol use, or smoking, then he or she will be willing to acknowledge depression and seek help.

If the simple acknowledgment of the depression is not enough to get the person motivated, then usually I recommend a visit with our medical social worker, a psychologist, or a psychiatrist. I often make the initial referral directly to the psychiatrist. As I said earlier about the importance of making a person's symptoms even a little better right away, so that he or she feels something can be done to help, the same applies to the treatment of depression—once acknowledged or recognized, something needs to be done as soon as possible to get a person headed in the right direction. Often, I find the psychiatrist most willing to start antidepressant medication that does help so much of the time. Most of the newer antidepressant medications block serotonin reuptake in the brain and are usually safer for heart patients than some of the older medications. Even elderly patients, and I really should say, especially elderly patients, can tolerate these medications and feel better psychologically.

Recently, there has been a lot of news in the lay press about the use of St. John's Wort for the treatment of depression, and because it was touted as a "natural" remedy, many of my patients felt they could take it without getting my advice. Well, I must say that several of them did respond nicely to the medication, and from what I have seen so far, there has been little in the way of adverse experiences.

In summary, I began this chapter by talking about how the mind can affect the body and concluded by talking about how the body can affect the mind. An awful lot of lip service is given to the term *holistic* care, but I believe that addressing all of the issues of mind and body only makes good sense in terms of the goals of improving the status of heart failure patients and their families.

5

Doctor-Patient Relationships:
How to Find and Work with the Right Physicians

I can't begin to tell you how much comment there has been about this chapter—and mostly positive. We are certainly undergoing a great deal of change in health care in our country: not only change in terms of how health care is delivered and paid for, but also a major shift in the types of diseases that are affecting people in general. Rather than acute diseases playing a major role, such as heart attack, pneumonia, and so on, the chronic diseases such as arthritis, diabetes, emphysema, and heart failure are affecting more and more patients.

This shift toward a "chronic disease mentality" means that a doctor not only has to have the skills needed to take care of emergent situations but also the skills, personality, and inclination to take care of a patient, and often some of the family, on a more chronic, recurring basis.

Patients' interactions with their doctors can have a tremendous impact on their treatment and quality of life. Although this statement is true for any illness, it is especially relevant for heart failure patients and their physicians because of the disease's chronicity. Because patients with heart failure rarely have just a once-a-year checkup, they need the kind of relationship with their physician that can endure the ups and downs, periods of feeling better and periods of feeling worse. There may be multiple office visits but, I hope, few hospital visits. Therefore, a good relationship between patient and physician is crucial. In many ways, this relationship is much like a good marriage: It must be prepared for the long haul and must be based on mutual appreciation, trust, working together, honesty, and, most of all, communication. Poor communication in this disease can mean the difference between success and failure.

My goal in this chapter is to provide patients with the information they require to choose the right physician, be alert to difficulties in the patient-physician relationship, and identify their own responsibilities. I want to show them how to get the best treatment they possibly can by establishing good communication with their doctor. To help you understand how all this can be accomplished, I'm going to walk you through the process that takes place when a person is first diagnosed with heart failure.

FIRST CONTACT

In this country, only 17 percent of all patients with heart failure get their care from a cardiologist. *And this is how it should be!* Since heart failure is so common, the majority of patients are cared for by primary care doctors (doctors in family practice, general practice, or internists). Many heart failure patients enter the system complaining to their primary care physician about such seemingly vague symptoms as fatigue, lethargy, and shortness of breath.

Doctors typically respond in a variety of ways, depending on how they interpret the symptoms and the findings of the examination. They may start with blood tests that come back as normal. Frequently, doctors attribute symptoms to the aging process and do little else. Sometimes fluid congestion in the lungs is thought to be asthma or pneumonia. Even if there is a history of coronary disease in a patient, doctors frequently focus on the short-term goal of preventing a heart attack and ignore the long-term possibility of heart failure. In many instances, aging truly may be the sole cause of the symptoms, and in other cases, preventing a heart attack correctly should take priority over preventing heart failure. The problem, however, is that when heart failure symptoms are overlooked, misdiagnosed, or ignored, the patient suffers needlessly when there is so much that can be done today.

It's possible that your doctor has correctly diagnosed heart failure but is not doing everything possible to maximize your treatment. The question arises as to when you should ask to be referred to a cardiologist, a specialist in internal medicine who has received additional training in cardiovascular disease. I would say that, in general, you should consider contacting a cardiologist or ask to be referred to one if

- You don't respond to treatment, that is, if your symptoms don't improve or if they become worse, or if you have had multiple hospital admissions for heart failure.
- You're diagnosed with heart failure but your physician can't pinpoint the cause.

- You are at risk (see Chapter 2) and have symptoms you think may be related to heart failure, but heart failure has not been mentioned as a potential cause.
- You're increasingly limiting your activities because of heart failure.
- You've been diagnosed as having mild heart failure and perhaps are not taking any medications (our current thoughts are that even very early symptomatic patients benefit from some medical therapy).

CARDIOLOGISTS AND OTHER SPECIALISTS

All cardiologists are not alike, and simply seeing a cardiologist does not mean you will get better or more advanced heart failure care. It is interesting to see that, owing to the major increase in the incidence of heart failure and the need to reduce health care costs, heart failure is getting more and more attention by professionals, hospital administrators, news reporters, and politicians alike. I recall even a couple of years ago going to give grand rounds lectures on heart failure to physician groups of not more than eight or ten people (half of whom were asleep!). Now, interest has increased, there's better attendance, and frequently, there's a hospital administrator present. The questions go on forever! Nevertheless, since heart failure has been around forever, there is a general feeling that we know all there is to know already. That is why I feel treating heart failure is like an avocation—you either love treating heart failure or you don't. I feel that an interest in heart failure translates into more concern, more attention to detail, and better care.

The point is that cardiologists don't have a lock on interest in heart failure. In fact, I have seen terrific interest and skill in treating heart failure in recent years, having been exposed to some of the excellent primary care physicians in our community. A cardiologist whose interest is in something other than heart failure, such as catheterization or balloon angioplasty, may not be as aggressive in treating heart failure. Also, though professional journals, videos, and meetings provide a great deal of information on the newer treatments for heart failure, what is taken up and used is very dependent on interest. My advice, therefore, is to continue to search until you find a physician with an interest in you and an interest in heart failure. If your primary care doctor wants to refer you to a cardiologist, again, you should ask the same question: "Will the cardiologist have an interest in me, and does he or she have an interest in heart failure?"

It's also possible that other specialists will be involved in your treatment. Sometimes other organs or conditions become involved with heart failure. The following is a list of the specialists who are most likely to be called upon and why:

- Kidney specialists *(nephrologists)* may be asked to give advice on how to improve kidney function or even to do dialysis (cleaning of the blood by a machine). Kidney problems may be due to diabetes, drugs, aging, or even heart failure itself.
- Diabetes specialists *(endocrinologists)* may be consulted on how to better control diabetes, which commonly involves kidney and heart problems, including heart failure; often, better control of the diabetes can improve heart failure symptoms and vice versa.
- Lung specialists *(pulmonologists)* may be consulted because the heart and lungs really work as a single unit. Many patients have both heart failure and lung problems, such as emphysema, lung cancer, or pneumonia. Even more common, the heart can cause lung problems (wheezing, congestion), and at times, lung problems can directly affect the heart (right-sided heart failure or cor pulmonale).

SHOULDN'T EVERY HEART FAILURE PATIENT HAVE A HEART FAILURE SPECIALIST?

Heart failure patients don't necessarily need a heart failure specialist, and even when they do, it's not always possible to get one. Primary care physicians and cardiologists may do a fine job of taking care of heart failure patients, even if they're not specialists in heart failure. It all depends on their level of interest! If the cause of the failure is relatively easy to determine and treat, if the progress of the failure is slowed or arrested, and if the patient feels better, then a specialist probably isn't needed.

Too often, however, heart failure doesn't follow this ideal scenario. The cause can be difficult to track down, and effective treatment can require a fine balance of medications and other measures. Heart failure specialists, because of their training and experience, are in the best position to orchestrate all this. They're also probably in charge of an experimental drug or treatment research program, one that may prove helpful to patients who haven't responded to conventional treatment.

Unfortunately, there are relatively few true heart failure specialists in this country, that is, cardiologists who spend 100 percent of their time working with heart failure patients. In fact, if you ask your primary care doctor for a referral, he or she might not be able to provide one. In small towns, especially, you won't have much luck (you may even have difficulty finding a cardiologist). But even in major metropolitan areas, you might not have any luck. You may want to contact local hospitals that have heart transplant programs, but even at such hospitals there is no guarantee that you will find a dedicated heart failure specialist with access to new and investigational treatments. Remember, the key is understanding—if you cannot figure out what the doctor has said, try again or get another doctor!

DOCTOR-DOCTOR COMMUNICATION

Because more than one physician is usually involved in a heart failure patient's treatment, coordination of effort is imperative. If one doctor is unaware that another has changed a patient's medication, the result can be a potentially life-threatening situation. A delicate balance of medication, diet, and other factors is necessary, and although one physician should be in charge of maintaining that balance, all health care professionals need to work together effectively. Unfortunately, our electronic age has not yet made this any easier.

The primary care physician is often in the best position to oversee the patient's care, to act as the quarterback of the team, even if a heart failure specialist is involved. A family doctor can monitor treatment in light of the patient's history and is able to establish a baseline against which the patient's changing condition can be measured. He or she can also take care of secondary problems associated with heart failure—urinary tract infections, colds, diabetes—that cardiologists often are unable or unwilling to address. Finally, the primary care physician can provide a long-term perspective on the patient's prior medical conditions, home life, and other physical or emotional issues, as well as communicate with other doctors and family members, keeping everyone in the information loop regarding a change in the patient's treatment or condition. I cannot overemphasize the importance of a good primary care doctor; I personally insist that patients keep or try to establish a relationship with a family doctor.

DOCTORS' ROLES AND PATIENTS' ROLES

Whether you've chosen a cardiologist or a primary care doctor to treat your heart failure, that physician should be a combination of Sherlock Holmes and Ronald Reagan. In other words, he or she should be an excellent investigator and a good communicator.

One of my patients once told me, "I like you because you seem like you're a good detective." A detective is an appropriate analogy, since heart failure specialists must search and probe not only for the cause of the heart failure but also for the most effective treatment. Because there are so many different causes of the disorder and subtleties of treatment, a good heart failure physician is constantly looking for something revealing or for a new and better approach.

Communication, too, is a valuable commodity. I've found that what sometimes helps heart failure patients the most isn't a fancy drug or procedure but simply information. I've had patients who come to me complaining about how terrible they feel admit that they aren't limiting their salt or fluids. When I ask them why they aren't limiting these things, they respond, "My doctor never told me to." Doctors sometimes assume that patients know more than they do. Communicating clearly what patients should and should not do greatly facilitates treatment.

The doctor-patient relationship, however, isn't a one-way street. I'm always chagrined when I see patients who absolve themselves of responsibility for their treatment, who tell me they don't know which medications to take because their spouse or someone else always tells them. Psychologically and physiologically, patients benefit from assuming responsibility not only for their medications but also for as many aspects of their treatment as possible. They should ask for an explanation of an unexpected new symptom and should proactively tell their doctors when another doctor changes their medication.

Patients should come prepared when they meet with their doctors. That means making sure the doctor has all medical records or can gain access to them, bringing their medications with them to their appointments, and keeping a diary of medications taken and symptoms noticed.

Adapting to each other's interpersonal style is a project for the patient and the physician. For instance, my style is to talk to patients, examine them, write some notes, review previous records, think intensely about their problems and decide what else to do or try, and then discuss my decisions with them. At the end of the office visit, I ask if there are further questions and make sure they don't need any prescription refills. Until patients figure out my style, they think I will bolt out of the room before they get a question answered or a prescription written. So, inevitably, they keep on talking when I'm doing my thinking. After a few visits and my explaining about my thinking period, I am accorded more silence. (It's funny how silence in a doctor's office is very uncomfortable for most people.) Other details, such as the best time to call the doctor or to ask questions during an examination or how to schedule appointments and get prescription refills are a matter of getting used to each other.

HEART FAILURE PATIENTS' QUESTIONS

One of the most important things a patient can do is to come armed with a list of questions. Too often, patients leave the doctor's office without getting the answers they need. To prevent this, I've created two lists of questions to share with you. The first contains questions heart failure patients most frequently ask, and the second list has questions that are often on their minds but aren't asked either because they're too embarrassed to ask them or because they're not sure how to articulate them. Because of the uniqueness of each patient's situation, no answers to these questions are offered here. Instead, the lists are meant as a introduction to dialogue between patient and doctor.

Most Frequently Asked Questions

- When can I return to certain activities (for example, sports)?
- When can I go back to work?
- What activities, foods, and other things do I have to limit?
- Should I exercise and, if so, how much?
- Can I have sex?
- Can I take my water pill early in the day?
- What is the intended effect of this medication?
- What side effects should I expect?
- Why is this test being done?
- What are the alternatives to this medication (or test)?
- What should I do if I forget or skip a medication?

Unasked Questions That Should Be Asked

- Am I doing myself harm when I get short of breath?
- How will my condition affect my sex life?
- How long am I going to live?
- Is this disease transmittable to my children?
- Is this given procedure going to hurt?
- Does my insurance cover this procedure (or drug)?

There are many more questions for each list, depending on the patient and his or her particular situation. Whatever the questions are, you should make sure you pose them to your doctor. Write a list at home and take it with you. No matter how stupid or embarrassing some of them might seem, don't be afraid to ask. Not only are the answers important for the heart failure patient's mental well-being, but also the questions enable patients to communicate their concerns to their doctor. I have actually seen a feeling of great calm come over my most anxious patients who come in with a long list of questions; as we go through the list and answer each question, the patients realize they are being listened to and understood.

SUMMARY

In summary, there is no absolute right doctor to care for your heart failure, but the doctor should be someone with more than a passing interest in heart failure. If you're not making progress or are even getting worse, ask your doctor for a referral or seek out a specialist. Remember, you will, I hope, have a very long-term relationship with whoever cares for your heart failure. Also, since you may have to rely on him or her to help you with very serious decisions (taking experimental drugs, undergoing surgery, going on kidney dialysis, or getting a heart transplant), pick a good communicator as well. Be a good communicator in return, and allow yourselves time to learn each other's individual style. Those are critical steps toward success with heart failure.

6

Heart Attacks and Heart Failure:
What's the Difference?

People frequently confuse coronary disease (blocked arteries that can lead to heart attacks) and heart attacks with heart failure. Either they use the terms synonymously or they inextricably link them. Although coronary disease is a common pathway to heart failure, it does not always lead to it. Obviously, you can have heart failure without ever having had a heart attack. To make the connections and distinctions clear, I will examine coronary disease's impact on the heart muscle.

"TIME IS MUSCLE"

When arteries are blocked with cholesterol and blood platelets, little or no blood flows through the artery to the heart muscle. When the muscle doesn't receive blood, chest pain, also known as *angina,* results. When such pain is prolonged, it usually means that serious damage is being done to the heart muscle and, if not quickly reversed, a heart attack will ensue. This prolonged period of pain is the prelude to a heart attack, since blood is being denied to the heart muscle. The sooner the blockage is cleared with a clot-busting drug, a catheter, or a balloon, the less the damage to the muscle and the lower the risk of a heart attack (thus, one drug company's slogan: "Time is muscle").

The more damage done to the heart muscle, either through repeated tiny attacks of angina or from one or more heart attacks, the more likely it is that the patient will experience heart failure. Though it's difficult to pinpoint the exact amount of damage that guarantees the progression to heart failure, most doctors agree that around 40 percent (that is, 40 percent of the left ventricle, which is the main pumping chamber of the heart) is the point of no return. The percentage is cumulative: It does not matter whether it's 40 percent damage from one heart attack or 25 percent from the first, 5 percent from the second, and 10 percent from a third. So it's possible for the interval between a person's first heart attack and the beginning of heart failure to be months or even years; the person might not reach the 40 percent figure until a third or fourth heart attack.

The 40 percent damage might come not just from the actual heart attack. Often multiple or repeated attacks of angina can cause heart failure. There are other factors that in combination with a relatively mild heart attack can push people into the heart failure category, including the following:

- Diabetes mellitus
- High blood pressure
- Prolonged angina episodes (Such episodes can scar the heart muscle.)
- Medications (Examples of drugs that may have a negative effect on heart muscle function are verapamil, metoprolol, and flecaninide.)
- Bypass surgery (The problem is that bypass grafts can close over time, without doctors or patients realizing they've closed. This can be a painless process causing a silent heart attack, which still weakens the heart muscle. Since the majority of bypass grafts close within ten years of the procedure, this is a common problem.)

LIMIT THE DAMAGE

Heart attacks don't have to progress to heart failure. If you can keep the damage under 40 percent, you can postpone or avoid failure. To do so, however, requires a keen awareness that you're not out of the woods simply because you survived a heart attack. In many instances, a bypass or other procedure and drugs may cause you to feel great, and your heart function may be excellent. You feel so good that you start repeating the behaviors that caused your heart attack—smoking, drinking, a high-fat diet, no exercise, stressful activities. Then you have another heart attack, but this time the muscle is damaged beyond the 40 percent limit and heart failure symptoms develop.

Until recently, doctors focused on helping patients overcome the acute condition of a heart attack but did not have reliable means for helping to prevent the development of heart failure. Many times, this translated into the wrong choice of medications: Drugs were given to patients that actually weakened their heart (but relieved the pain associated with coronary disease). Or physicians recommended no medications for patients who had relatively minor heart attacks. But a recent study shows that even people who have suffered small heart attacks experience heart enlargement if they don't receive appropriate medication. Enlargement weakens the heart and increases the chances of failure. Early use of these medicines (for example, captopril) may prevent or delay the development of heart failure for many heart attack victims and may even decrease the amount of damage.

Lowering the Percentage of Damage

One of the great discoveries made by Dr. Dean Ornish and other cardiologists is that coronary disease can be reversed. This is good news for coronary disease victims and even better news for prospective heart failure patients. If you've experienced 20 or 30 percent damage to your heart muscle, you're perilously close to heart failure. But if you can reduce the risk of another heart attack, you've taken a big step back from the precipice.

Also, the thinking goes that if 20 percent of the muscle is damaged, perhaps half of that, or 10 percent, is not irreversibly damaged but is, instead, "hibernating." That is, the metabolism of the heart has slowed because it isn't receiving sufficient blood; it has become very "quiet" in order to protect itself. But if you restore the blood flow, this 10 percent can "wake up" and be healthy muscle again. We've found that even if a patient experiences 40 percent damage, some of that damaged muscle function can be restored.

The key, therefore, is to remove blockages and start blood flowing to the heart as quickly as possible after the heart attack. A cardiologist recently told me that he was doing an electrocardiogram (EKG) on a patient at the hospital when the patient experienced huge changes in the EKG, signaling a heart attack. The cardiologist immediately moved the patient to the heart catheterization lab; the artery where the blockage was seen was identified and the blockage was removed. Three days later, this patient underwent an aggressive exercise test, and his heart function was perfectly normal; what damage there was had been minimized or quickly reversed, and the patient's risk of heart failure was greatly reduced.

One good piece of news is that for most heart attack victims two medicines are routinely used—these are ACE inhibitors and beta-blockers (see Chapter 8). Indeed, many hospitals are monitored on how frequently their patients who have had a heart attack get these medicines. As it turns out, these medicines, which seem to allow the heart to heal better and prevent other heart attacks, are also two of the key medicines we use to treat heart failure. So making sure you get on the right medications after a heart attack and staying on them may be a good first step in preventing a future of heart failure.

DETERMINING YOUR RISK

Ischemic heart disease, or heart attack, is one of the worst pathways to heart failure. Compared to other heart failure patients, those with a history of heart attacks generally have a poorer prognosis, feel worse, and are more likely to succumb to sudden death. Typically, these patients are also more vulnerable to arrhythmia (irregular heartbeats) than other patients.

Given all this, it's important to do everything possible after a heart attack to determine your risk for another one. Although that second attack may not do as much damage as the first, and you may survive it, the cumulative damage could nudge you into heart failure. Before you leave the hospital, therefore, your cardiologist should "stratify" your risk for a subsequent heart attack. This can be done by using a variety of tests, including an echocardiogram and Holter, MUGA, and treadmill tests, as well as by determining what kind of heart attack you had. In addition, patients who complain of chest pain after the initial attack tend to be more vulnerable than others.

If you're at high risk for another heart attack, your doctor should be aggressive in his or her treatment, that is, in finding and removing blockages, prescribing appropriate medications, and designing strict diet and exercise regimens. Since there is a common link between heart attacks and heart failure, aggressively limiting the severity of damage done to the heart by coronary artery disease can help to weaken that connection and possibly sever it.

UNDERSTANDING YOUR RISK:
WHAT ABOUT HOMOCYSTEINE?

Applicable to this topic of heart attack and vascular diseases in general, such as stroke and poor circulation to the limbs (what we call peripheral vascular disease), is the relative risk factors for these diseases. By now, I hope most people are aware of what we call the traditional risk factors for coronary artery disease. These include

- Age
- Male sex (at least until the menopause for women)
- Cigarette smoking
- High blood pressure
- Sedentary lifestyle
- Obesity
- High cholesterol and other blood lipids
- Diabetes mellitus

- Family history (another family member who had premature or early development of coronary artery disease)

Usually, when we see patients who have had a heart attack or we are trying to sort out their risk and advise them, we look to these kinds of factors. However, we all know people who have had none of these factors and still have a heart attack. Years ago, one of my mentors used to comment that the average cholesterol for a patient hospitalized with a heart attack was less than 210 mg/dl. His point was that we consider "normal" at too high a level. However, perhaps cholesterol or smoking or high blood pressure wasn't the entire explanation.

In the last few years, scientists have discovered a genetic disease in which there is an elevation of the homocysteine levels in the blood, which causes an increased incidence of vascular problems. Homocysteine is an amino acid, the stuff of which our body proteins are made. High levels have been associated not only with heart and blood vessel disease but also with eye problems, bone problems, and even psychological problems. Interestingly, not only can elevated levels of homocysteine arise from genetic causes but also diseases that cause abnormal production or metabolism of the amino acid and its metabolic pathway. These include

- Chronic renal failure
- Leukemia
- Psoriasis
- Hypothyroidism
- Vitamin deficiencies (folic acid, B_6 and B_{12}—see treatment below)
- Drugs (examples are methotrexate and seizure medications)

One of the good pieces of news coming out of this new information about the possibility that homocysteine may be another important risk factor is that the treatment is relatively simple and inexpensive. Usually, replacement of folic acid with or without vitamins B_6 and B_{12} is sufficient to reduce the levels of homocysteine. The exact doses are not yet known, but I usually recommend at least 400 micrograms per day of folic acid (about four times the usual minimal recommended daily allowance). I would strongly recommend that you discuss this issue with your doctor if you are concerned about coronary artery disease or vascular disease.

In summary, the relationship between heart attack and heart failure is a close one, but the two are not the same. If you still do not understand this important difference, then I'd suggest you reread this chapter or ask your doctors and nurses to explain it to you.

7

Conventional Treatments for Heart Failure

Like all things in life, when discussing the treatment of heart failure, there are certain core elements or the "basics" that I feel should be considered or discussed with most patients. This does not mean that all of these treatments should be or will be used, but depending on each patient's situation, these are the building blocks of treatment for most patients.

Therefore, in this chapter, I would like to outline some of the conventional or standard treatments for heart failure that are being used today. These are common procedures or medications that can or should be applied to most people who have heart failure. Obviously, how many of these treatments are applied to any one individual depends on the seriousness of his or her heart failure. In addition to the prescribed medications, other treatments, such as dietary restrictions, can and should be explained thoroughly, if not by the doctor, then by the nurses, dietitians, or office staff involved with caring for the patient.

SALT RESTRICTION

I recently saw a middle-aged gentlemen who had come to see me at the recommendation of another cardiologist. After I had taken the initial part of his history, it was clear that the patient had a fairly advanced case of heart failure. A quick glance at the medications he was taking indicated that his fine cardiologist had already given him most of the conventional medications he should have had. The patient had been through an elaborate series of tests, and every bit of information to be known about his diagnosis had already been determined. Finally, I turned to the patient and his wife and began to ask them about sources of sodium that might be in his diet. With heart failure, the heart's ability to pump blood is impaired, and the body senses this as not having enough blood in the circulation (see the section on diuretics later in this chapter). This stimulates the body to retain salt, with the goal of retaining even more fluid. Obviously, then, eliminating salt in the diet is one of the first steps in helping to reduce the excess fluid that may accumulate in the body. In fact, when we discuss diuretics, or water pills, you will see that their primary task is to clear salt out of the body and then the water that tends to follow.

This patient at some point had been told to restrict the salt in his diet, but he had not been given detailed instructions about this. He told me that he did not add any extra salt from the saltshaker, but when I reviewed several of his favorite meals, it became clear that he was getting loads of salt in seemingly innocent ways. For example, one of his favorite treats was to go to a local restaurant where they had "home-cooked soup and a terrific salad bar." What more could a cardiologist ask for? he thought. Unfortunately, the tasty homemade soup was loaded with salt, and the patient did not realize that the salad bar that looked so great was sprayed with a sodium-containing preservative to help keep those fruits and vegetables looking fresh. And his favorite house dressing would have sent the salt police into a tizzy! Additionally, all of the canned vegetables he was using were high in salt, and he was unaware of the high salt content in most of his other condiments. The final blow came when he told me about some frozen dinners he frequently consumed, all under a terrifically healthy-sounding name, but when I went and got a sample box for him to look at, it turned out that practically every meal contained 1,000 milligrams of salt, more than half of what his total daily intake of salt should have been (see Chapter 11). One of our heart failure nurses spent forty-five minutes with the patient and his wife instructing them on how to pick foods with a lower sodium content. I think it came as a tremendous shock to them that despite all the husband's medical therapy, his treatment was inadequate because he was not controlling the salt in his diet, something that was well within his power. When I saw this patient about two weeks later, he was feeling remarkably better, yet I really hadn't done a thing to treat him.

Sodium restriction, then, is critical. The degree of restriction is individualized, but I generally tell my patients not to exceed two grams of salt a day. Unless you are used to eating heavily salted foods, this in fact is fairly liberal, and you can learn to enjoy food with this sodium restriction. Basically, I follow the two-gram limit because that is what most patients learn in the hospital; also, if I tell them more than two grams, they tend to exceed that limit, anyway. I tend to be a little less strict with patients who do not have a serious problem with fluid retention, but I do insist on some sodium restriction for virtually everyone. The following analogy illustrates the point I'm making here: If you are going to build a beautiful home, it makes no sense to put thousands of dollars into building and decorating it unless you have a solid foundation. The same applies to treating patients with heart failure: Patients can be on every drug in the book, as well as on every experimental medication, but their heart failure won't get better unless they adhere to the basic rules, which include salt and fluid restriction. All too often, I think we doctors assume that patients are getting specific information about salt restriction from either the nurses or the dietitians, and that may or may not be true. Furthermore, although patients have been told about salt restriction in the past, they need to hear it again and again, and in commonsense terms. One patient told me that he was aware that he was supposed to be on a two-gram sodium diet, but then his next question was, "What is a gram?" Patients are frequently too embarrassed or intimidated to ask for specific information, but they must have this information. There is a wide variety of good information out there, in books, magazines, and publications available from your local chapter of the American Heart Association.

Finally, patients always ask me about salt substitutes. By and large, I think that these are acceptable, but you have to be careful, because some of the salt substitutes are, in fact, potassium salts instead of sodium salts. Very high levels of potassium in the diet can be as serious a problem as high levels of sodium. My best advice is this: Learn to eat a restricted sodium diet, and you and your heart failure will be better for it.

I recently read an article from another country extolling the benefit of salt. However, I think that anyone who has a perfectly normal cardiac situation can handle and get rid of excess salt taken in the diet. This is the concept of homeostasis—that is to say, no matter how hard we try to throw off Mother Nature, the natural tendency is to restore homeostasis and try to maintain the normal levels and functions of the body. A good example of homeostasis is how we generally keep our body temperature constant despite being exposed to a wide variety of outside temperatures.

In short, when it comes to salt . . . Just Don't Do It!

FLUID RESTRICTION

Yet another cornerstone in the treatment of heart failure is fluid restriction. Again, since one of the primary problems with heart failure is excess fluid in the body, which the heart must pump to the kidneys to get it out of the body, then it makes sense that the smaller the volume of fluid going in, the less work there is for the weakened heart and the less congestion there will be in the body. However, I think it is common to find patients with severe heart failure and who take all kinds of medications, but who have never once been told to restrict the fluids in their diet. In fact, when I ask patients about restricting fluids, I've had many quite proudly announce, "Oh no, doctor, I try to drink as much water as I can each day!" I think we have all heard since childhood that it is wise to drink plenty of fluids. Unfortunately, I must tell patients that this is terrific advice as long as they don't have heart failure. Once they understand that they need to restrict fluids, controlling heart failure is often amazingly simplified.

The same sorts of problems come up with fluid restriction as with salt restriction: Since there are multiple hidden sources of fluid, we try to make sure that patients count the fluid in their soups, juices, coffee, tea, and soft drinks— even the water they drink to help them swallow their pills (some patients who have heart failure take so many pills that this can be a considerable source of fluid). Once again, the amount of fluid restriction depends on the individual case, but by and large, we tell most patients to limit fluid consumption to one to two quarts a day.

Some patients need to be more strict than others, and for some, the two quarts can be liberalized. My experience is that most patients tend to underestimate how much fluid they actually drink. Many patients who come to see me with refractory heart failure end up on the same medications that were prescribed for them before—or even on less medication—simply by becoming believers in fluid restriction. We've had success with many different methods of keeping track of this two-quart limit, but perhaps none is as successful as the following system, which a patient of mine invented. Basically, at the beginning of each day he filled up a two-quart container with water. Each time he drank some fluid, he poured the same amount of fluid out of the container. He told me that when the container was empty, he stopped drinking for the day.

Perhaps the most severe complaint I get from my patients who go on fluid restriction is that their mouths are dry. This, of course, is due to the fluid restriction as well as the water pills they are already taking. If your doctor feels you can do with a little more fluid or a little less diuretic, appropriate adjustments can be made. There are many tricks I teach my patients so that they can learn to live with the fluid restriction and thereby live better with their heart failure. Some of the things I commonly recommend to my patients to help them keep their mouths moist and maintain fluid restriction are the following: chewing gum, popsicles, sucking ice cubes or chips, small sips of water (instead of big gulps!), and hard candies. Frequently brushing your teeth is also helpful.

Now, many patients and even other doctors have told me that they think the concept of fluid restriction is wrong. There is some basis, or should I say bias, for this line of reasoning. In animals and even in people who have normal hearts, if the fluid intake is severely restricted, it will cause the body to secrete a hormone called renin (see previous chapters). This renin helps to do several normally good things, including stimulate the thirst sensors in the brain to try and tell us to find and drink water. However, renin can also cause stimulation of some of the neuro-hormones and indirectly cause even more dysfunction of the heart muscle. However, in general, people who are taking diuretics or water pills for heart failure already have this mechanism of renin secretion turned on, and limiting water is not going to be the inciting factor. Continuous use of powerful diuretics, with their effect on the calcium in the bones, the losses of potassium and magnesium, and so on, are far more important risks. Again, you have to use common sense, but I believe that for most patients, fluid restriction makes good sense!

CONVENTIONAL DRUG THERAPIES

For many years, doctors have relied on a couple of simple medications to help control the symptoms of heart failure. Although the treatments used for many other diseases in medicine have changed dramatically from those used fifty or 100 years ago, many of the heart failure treatments have remained the same. The primary reason for this is that these treatments do work, at least in terms of relieving some of the symptoms of patients with heart failure.

The three common drugs considered the core treatment for the heart failure patient today are the diuretics, or water pills; digoxin; and a group of medicines called angiotensin-converting enzyme inhibitors, or ACE inhibitors. Digoxin has been used for hundreds of years, whereas the clinical use of ACE inhibitors has only spanned the last ten years. Interestingly, there is more clinical information proving the safety and efficacy of the ACE inhibitors than there is for diuretics and digoxin. Nonetheless, the use of drugs such as diuretics and digoxin are so ingrained in the treatment of a patient with heart failure that virtually every patient who needs them is put on them routinely. Unfortunately, this is not always the case for ACE inhibitors. Perhaps because they are relatively new, or because of a doctor's lack of familiarity with recent medical studies on ACE inhibitors, it is estimated that between 40 and 70 percent of patients who should be on these drugs are not! In the following paragraphs, I discuss a little bit of the rationale for the use of each of these agents, including some of the pros and cons your doctor will weigh when deciding whether to use these medications for you. Perhaps the biggest advance in medical therapy since ACE inhibitors is elevation of the beta-blockers (Coreg or carvedilol, Toprol XL or metoprolol, and Zebeta or bisopro-lol) to standard therapy. I am so excited about this for several reasons. First, this is one of the first drug therapies to significantly add to the life-saving abilities of the ACE inhibitors; yes, I did say life saving. It is now proven that these medications make people with heart failure feel better and at the same time begin to improve the ejection fraction as well as to help keep patients alive and out of the hospital.

The other reason I am so excited is that my early research interests were in the use of beta-blockers in heart failure. Over fifteen years ago we were trying these medications even though most doctors laughed or even scorned us for doing so. I am happy we had the fortitude to stick to what we thought made good sense.

Aside from the diuretics, digoxin, ACE inhibitors, and beta-blockers, we continue to try and investigate new drugs to improve on what is available. A lesson we have learned is that we are not always so successful. Recently, using drugs that lower catecholamines (monoxidine) or drugs that block TNF alpha, we have thought we were adding a way to impact the abnormal neurohormones released into a person's body. Unfortunately, these trials have not proven that these approaches are helpful and so investigation goes on.

Another group of drugs, which act similarly to the ACE inhibitors, are called A2RBs (Angiotensin II receptor blockers). Although they lack some of the ACE inhibitor side effects, such as cough, they really are not equivalent to an ACE inhibitor.

One idea was to try adding an ACE inhibitor and an A2RB for a beneficial effect—this was tested in a large trial that seemed to show that the combination did reduce hospitalizations but did not reduce mortality any more than the ACE inhibitor alone. Therefore, simply put, an ACE inhibitor and a beta-blocker are standard heart failure therapy, usually combined with digoxin and a diuretic if the patient is retaining fluid. I discuss each of these drugs in a little more detail below.

The A II receptor blockers (Cozaar or losartan, or Diovan or valsartan, or Avapro or irbesartan) also block the effect of A II on the cells in a way that is different from the ACE inhibitors. Because the A II receptor blockers don't cause the side effect of cough as often as the ACE inhibitors, there has been a ready change to using them as a first-line drug. Unfortunately, we do not yet have the same survival studies on these drugs, so the role of these drugs remains unknown in part. Interestingly, ongoing studies combine the use of an ACE inhibitor and an A II receptor blocker to see if they have a synergistic effect. I hope we'll know more over the next several years about the role of these drugs in conventional heart failure treatments.

DIURETICS

To understand why we use diuretics in treating patients with heart failure, you must first understand one of the important ways in which the body responds to a decrease in heart function. During our evolution we have carried with us the so-called homeostatic mechanisms, which are reactions that help keep our biological processes as stable as possible. Our bodily homeostatic mechanisms were probably developed to respond not to heart failure but, rather, to sudden losses in blood flow, for example, from having been attacked by a prehistoric carnivore. What the body, primarily the kidneys, then senses is that not enough blood is getting to it, and it sets in motion, in an attempt to restore the body to stability, a series of events that cause the body to avidly retain salt and fluids.

Unfortunately, when a person has heart failure and not enough blood flow gets to the kidneys, the same mechanism is set into action, and fluid and salt are again avidly retained. This is one of the first steps in setting up the vicious cycle of heart failure: The increase in fluid and salt in the body only serve to weaken the heart even further, which in turn decreases the blood flow to the kidneys even more, which means that more fluid and salt are retained, and so on.

Diuretics, or water pills, simply address the problem we have just discussed; that is, with heart failure, the patient retains excess fluid and salt, which overload the blood vessels, organs, and tissues of the entire body. Water pills attempt to clear the extra salt and water through the kidneys and thus rid the body of some of the extra fluid that it is retaining. Now, this is not quite as simple as it sounds. Water pills are prescribed for a variety of situations; for example, they are one of the commonly recommended treatments for high blood pressure as well as for the fluid retention many women encounter in the premenstrual period. In such settings, where the patient has normal heart function along with normal kidney function, the diuretic can frequently produce a "super" effect (and those who have taken a diuretic know what I mean; you feel as though you are spending the entire day in the bathroom!). For many patients with heart failure, however, the results are not the same: If the heart function is too weak to deliver enough blood flow to the kidneys, the diuretic's action may be minimal or absent. Therefore, there has to be at least some preserved cardiac pumping function in order to get the blood flow to the kidneys, so that the kidneys can create urine adequately; only then can a water pill aid the kidneys and help clear the excess fluid.

Another problem is that kidney function may already be impaired; frequently, the kidneys are operating at only 15 to 25 percent of normal. This may be due to many years of heart failure, where there was impaired blood flow to the kidneys, or to an underlying disease such as longstanding high blood pressure or diabetes mellitus, which may be in part responsible for the heart failure as well. In that situation, the effectiveness of the water pill will be diminished, and increasingly larger doses of water pills have to be used. When patients retain fluid and have leg edema, or leg swelling, they are actually retaining fluid everywhere in the body, including the lining of the stomach and the intestines. We forget that when we take a pill, it has to go down to the stomach and intestines and be absorbed through the linings of these organs and work its way into the bloodstream before it can ever do its job. Excess fluid in the lining of the stomach and intestines prevents or decreases the absorption of many medications, including water pills themselves. Some patients will notice that their water pills seem to work exceedingly well on certain days and less well or not at all on other days; this has a lot to do not only with the amount of blood flow to the stomach and intestines but also with the amount of swelling in the lining of those organs. When water pills taken by mouth produce no effect, the patient needs either to be seen in the office or hospitalized in order to get an intravenous dose of the diuretic medication, which goes right into the bloodstream and bypasses the absorption phase.

Nevertheless, oral water pills are one of the basic medications we employ, to a greater or lesser degree, in most patients who have some form of heart failure. In certain forms of heart failure (for example, in diastolic dysfunction, such as hypertrophic cardiomyopathy, or in forms of valvular heart problems, such as aortic stenosis), diuretics should be used with caution or not at all, since they can worsen the situation rather than improve it. The general trend is to give increasingly larger doses of diuretics as heart failure progresses, but other medications can be added to help limit these dosages.

There are a number of common side effects that occur with diuretics (see Chapter 8). Although their intended purpose is to help wash out some of the blood salts and minerals along with excess water, they can do so overzealously in some patients, which may result in dehydration as well as in severe electrolyte deficiencies (such as sodium, potassium, or magnesium), which in and of themselves can cause symptoms and can put the patient at increased risk for irregular heartbeats and worse heart function. Aside from causing electrolyte abnormalities, diuretics can wash out calcium, which can lead to weakened bones and precipitate deposits of uric acid into the joints, which can cause an attack of gout. Because of these potential problems, it is frowned on to have patients regulate the amount of diuretic medication they take by themselves.

By and large, the benefits diuretics produce outweigh the potential side effects, and most patients usually feel better when the excess fluid in their body has been cleared away. The use of diuretics has to be explained carefully to patients so that they understand what the medication is supposed to do and to not interpret the excess urination as an undesired effect. It is important to get an idea of what the patient's day is like and to try to schedule the diuretic doses around the person's daily routine. For example, if a person has an hour's train ride to work each morning, with no washroom facilities on the train, taking the diuretic first thing in the morning might not be the wisest choice. Similarly, if diuretics need to be taken twice a day and the patient waits until bedtime to take the second dose, he or she can forget about a good night's sleep. Sleep deprivation just leads to a vicious cycle of agitation, insomnia, and perhaps even serious changes in a person's disposition and mood. That is why I usually recommend that the second dose of the day, when needed, be taken just after the patient returns home from work in the afternoon. That gives the diuretic time to do its work and leaves patients more "dried out," if you will, so that they can get a good night's sleep. It is not uncommon for me to find within the first week or so of beginning treatment with a patient that simply rearranging medications to fit the lifestyle allows the patient his or her first good night's sleep in several years. A doctor's ignorance of a patient's routine can frequently lead to lots of missed doses of a diuretic, with the patient remaining edematous and symptomatic, and the doctor concluding that nothing more can be done for the patient. Usually, a happy medium can be achieved, so that the diuretic doses are taken and patients do not totally disrupt their lifestyle.

A word should be said about an older medication called Aldactone, or spironolactone. This used to be used as a relatively weak diuretic alone or in combination with other diuretics. Then, because of the stronger oral diuretics that became available, the use of spironolactone became less common. However, since this medication blocks one of the abnormal hormones (aldosterone), it was studied again and for patients with advanced heart failure, at least, it also seems to reduce the risk of death. So now again, we add small doses of this medication in addition to the other. One side effect that may limit its use in certain people is the development of enlarged or painful breast tissue, call gynecomastia. This seems most bothersome in men. Some newer medications that work the same without causing the side effects are still being studied.

The bottom line in using diuretics is for the patient to understand what the goals are and what side effects, both potentially serious as well as seemingly trivial, this kind of medication can produce, and for the doctor to prescribe the diuretics in a way that ensures their optimal use in the patient.

DIGOXIN

Digoxin is a medicine that has been available for over 200 years. Yet, surprisingly, we are still learning how it works in heart failure and what its potential advantages are. It has been used primarily for two main purposes in treating patients with heart failure. Digoxin acts within the heart muscle to improve its contraction and therefore the pumping action of the heart. Digoxin is also commonly used in patients who have irregular heartbeats, such as atrial fibrillation, which can cause the heart to beat too fast; that is, digoxin can slow the heartbeat or even help it become more regular.

Although digoxin is a very old drug, this does not necessarily mean that it is a completely safe one; in fact, side effects from it are fairly common. In the use of digoxin, we say that there is a narrow "therapeutic window," which means that the dosage has to be adjusted very carefully; if too little is given, there is no effect, and a little too much can actually cause bad effects and make a patient even worse. Probably because of the need to carefully adjust the dosage, as well as the lack of any study demonstrating that digoxin has a favorable effect on the mortality rate in heart failure, this drug has had a slight decline in popularity over the past ten years. However, two recent studies found that heart failure patients who were taken off digoxin for purposes of the study suffered a major decline in how they felt, and that more patients required hospitalization for recurrent bouts of heart failure. A large study sponsored by the National Institutes of Health showed that digoxin does not impact the mortality rate in patients with heart failure. However, we do know it often improves how they feel.

I think in many ways we are getting smarter about knowing when to use digoxin as well as when to be cautious in its use. For example, since much of the drug is cleared out of the body through the kidneys, people with poor kidney function, such as the elderly, may accumulate the drug and suffer more side effects. Also, since we can now more easily measure the level of digoxin in the blood, we can be alert to a high level and reduce the dose. Similarly, we find that some patients are taking a dose that is too low for them, and that simply increasing the dose can give them some help for their heart failure.

Unfortunately, digoxin interacts with many other drugs that are commonly used in heart failure. In fact, the absorption of digoxin can be altered by other drugs and even by the foods we eat. (The day after Oprah Winfrey had a guest on her television show explaining how certain foods affect the absorption of medicines, I got a rash of phone calls from patients who wanted to be sure I was aware of the fact that oat bran could significantly decrease the absorption of digoxin. I took this as a positive sign that many patients are taking more responsibility for their own health care.)

I think the important point to remember about digoxin is that although it is an old-fashioned remedy, it is commonly being used today in over 70 percent of patients with heart failure; up until about a decade ago, digoxin, along with diuretics, was truly the mainstay of therapy for patients with heart failure. I think in the next six years or so, we will learn a great deal more about this superb remedy for heart failure.

VASODILATORS AND ANGIOTENSIN-CONVERTING ENZYME INHIBITORS

The third core group of medicines used in treating patients with heart failure are vasodilators, or medicines that open up the arteries of the body to make the heart pumping function easier. I always tell patients that if you have a 1-horsepower motor pumping into a 1-inch tube or conduit, reducing the conduit to .5 inch is going to make the pump work even harder, whereas increasing the conduit to 1.5 inches is going to make the pump work more efficiently. That has been the basic idea behind the use of a variety of medications called vasodilators, which includes ACE inhibitors (ACEIs). When the body senses a decreased pumping action of the heart, it responds in a variety of ways to hold on to salt and water, but it also sends out chemical signals to narrow the arteries and veins of the body. This, too, is a homeostatic mechanism, with the goal of keeping the blood pressure stable, but in fact, it represents one of the processes that serves to worsen or accelerate a patient's heart failure, as application of the aforementioned analogy of the pump and conduit makes clear.

You might be surprised to learn that it was less than a decade ago that a clinical trial showed that a combination of vasodilators (hydralazine and isosorbide dinitrate) results in a reduction in mortality rate for patients with heart failure. Since then, more and more information has become available about the ACEIs, a new class of agents that actually block the production of one of the substances that causes the blood vessels to go into spasm or constrict. This class of drugs has been shown to be one of the most effective treatments for heart failure, not only in terms of reducing symptoms but also with respect to decreasing the mortality rate. In a clinical trial comparing the combination of hydralazine and isosorbide dinitrate with the ACEIs, the latter seem to have had a better effect on mortality rate. Drugs that fall within the ACEI category include captopril, enalapril, and lisinopril. There are still other drugs within this category that do not yet have specific approval for use in treating heart failure.

Despite the overwhelming evidence that these drugs are useful for treating patients with heart failure, it is estimated that perhaps only 25 to 40 percent of patients who should be on these drugs are actually taking them. There are some common side effects that can occur with the ACEIs that may cause the drugs to be discontinued in certain patients. Since these drugs open up the blood vessels, they can lower blood pressure, which may already be quite low in a patient with heart failure. They can also cause rashes and taste alteration (but these side effects are infrequent), as well as some worsening of the kidney function (again, this is infrequent and usually quickly reversible). On the other hand, they may improve kidney function in some patients, and that is why it is so important to try these drugs in most patients. One of the most common reasons patients stop taking these drugs, or why physicians remain reluctant to prescribe them, is that they can produce a cough. It has been estimated that the cough can occur in anywhere from 5 to 20 percent of patients, but my experience has been that much of the cough in patients with heart failure really is congestion or fluid in the lungs, and that once the patient is adequately "dried out," the cough is no longer a problem. There are new drugs being investigated and developed that work in a fashion similar to the ACEIs but that will bypass some of the adverse effects, such as the cough. Also, as was the case earlier with digoxin, we do not know the ideal dose of an ACEI for a patient to take. Again, within the next few years, we hope to have some better answers to our questions about these drugs.

The important point here is that these drugs have been shown to have such an important effect for heart failure patients that a serious attempt should be made to get most patients on these drugs while avoiding some of the side effects.

Beta-Blockers

As I said above, the understanding of the role of beta-blockers in heart failure has been one of the greatest advances for treating heart failure in the last ten years. These medications act to slow the heart rate and block the deleterious effect of neurohormones like the catecholamines. However, it is clear that these drugs work in many other ways as well. It is also clear that not all beta-blockers work in the same way and not all of them work for patients who have heart failure!

In using these drugs (Coreg or carvedilol, Toprol XL or metoprolol, and Zebeta or bisoprolol) there are several important things for you to know. The first is that doctors should start these drugs at very low doses and then slowly raise the doses over a period as long as two to three months. This makes sure that too much blockade is not given at any one time and that side effects can be monitored. Also, in some patients, even with very small doses the patient may feel a little more tired for the first few weeks of therapy; this is not a common side effect but one the patient should be prepared for so that they won't stop taking this important medicine. Often your doctor will need to adjust your other medicines and ACE inhibitor if your blood pressure gets too low, or the diuretic if you either begin to retain more fluid or get too dried out. We usually bring patients into our heart failure center to make these adjustments just so we can monitor the effects. Once patients begin to work up to slightly larger doses they begin to notice an improvement in how they feel.

Along with the improvement in overall well-being and a decrease in symptoms, beta-blockers also produce an improvement in the left ventricular ejection fraction and decrease the risk of death. All three of the beta-blockers have these effects and there are studies to support each of the three approved drugs. It seems that with carvedilol there is a wider range of doses that can provide improvements in survival and ejection fraction. There are certain special situations where your doctor may choose one medication over another.

The other thing to know about beta-blockers is that once on them you probably should not come off them, since withdrawal can definitely cause worsening. This happens when patients are admitted to the hospital. In general, if a patient gets worse and needs to be in the hospital several weeks or months after they have been stable on the beta-blockers, the reason for worsening is generally not related to the beta-blocker and it should *not* be discontinued. If, however, three or four days after a dose increase the person gets more symptoms, it might be reasonable to reduce the dose; I try to never take away the drug completely since it is so important.

We generally use these drugs for all patients with heart failure. Recent data also suggests that we can safely initiate small doses, even for patients with advanced heart failure and even for those in the hospital. Many heart failure experts also feel the earlier we use beta-blockers the better. Therefore, we also use them in patients with heart muscle weakness and no symptoms (asymptomatic ventricular dysfunction).

All in all, if you have heart failure you should either be on an ACE inhibitor *and* a beta-blocker *or know why not!*

SUMMARY

In this chapter, I have talked about some of the basic approaches to treating heart failure, including fluid and salt restriction and the use of core medicines. There are still many other drugs and treatments that could be considered conventional. For example, if a patient cannot tolerate one of the ACEI drugs, substituting the combination of hydralazine and isosorbide dinitrate would be a reasonable alternative and would still be considered a good conventional approach. In other chapters, we'll talk about some of the more advanced or investigational approaches to treating patients with heart failure. I want to emphasize, though, that unless a good foundation is established with conventional treatment, the more exotic investigational approaches are unlikely to succeed.

8

Summary of Common Heart Failure Drugs:

Indications, Doses, Side Effects, and Interactions with Other Drugs

Many years ago, when I was an intern, one of the wise residents who was helping me learn the art and science of medicine said, "Any drug can do anything." This simple saying has stood me in good stead over the years, and what it means is that in a given individual, any drug is capable of causing any type of side effect you could imagine. This is not uncommon—for example, so many people can drink milk or eat fish or strawberries, yet for some, these foods can cause a terrible reaction. In some, it causes rash; in others, cough; in still others, passing out.

Therefore, introducing any chemical substance into your body is a form of experiment. Usually, most of the experimenting has gone on in clinical trials before the drug is released, but there are always some early postmarket experiences with a new drug that were never detected in the large clinical research trials that preceded the drug's release. In fact, I know some doctors who won't prescribe a new drug until two years or more after its release by the FDA!

It is clear that even for patients who are not yet symptomatic, there is a role for drug therapy in virtually everyone who has heart failure. In fact, most patients with heart failure end up taking at least two medications. As we find out more about how these medications work and what impact they have on survival and outcome, heart failure patients will probably, at least for the next decade, end up taking more and more medications. It is well known that with each new medication, there is a risk of confusion regarding when it should be taken, what adverse side effects can be expected, and how it interacts with other drugs. (Appendix II lists resources for more information, including books that discuss in detail many of the side effects, indications, dosages, and so forth of each of the heart failure medications.)

I have long been aware of the cost of medications for heart failure patients. In fact, an inability to pay for some of the medications is not infrequently the reason a patient ends up back in the hospital with worsened heart failure. As I point out in a medical publication, the current average cost for just the core heart failure medications can easily approach over $1,000 each year. Although we are constantly reminded that the cost of drugs represents a small proportion of the cost of caring for patients with heart failure, it is unfortunately true that for most patients, the percentage of the cost of medication paid for by the patient is far greater than the percentage of hospitalization or office visit charges the patient must assume as out-of-pocket expenses. Because of patients' concerns about the cost of medication, I am frequently asked if generic and brand-name medications are equivalent. With few exceptions, I generally recommend that generics be provided for most of my patients. There are, however, a couple of circumstances where the bioavailability or absorption is better with the brand name than with the generic drug. This should be discussed with your physician. Similarly, there can be a wide range in the price of a medication, and I always encourage my patients to shop around, particularly with some of the more expensive medications. However, the pharmacy business has become quite competitive, and nowadays the large chains are often not significantly less expensive than your local pharmacist. I personally feel there is an important role to be played by the local pharmacist, and I think many patients turn to that individual for a lot of advice regarding their health care. In fact, a recent survey found that Americans still rank the local pharmacist as the most honorable and ethical professional.

Finally, let me emphasize how important it is to always carry with you a current list of your medications, including their dosages and how often you take them. This is critical whenever you visit a doctor, and if you are ever in an emergency situation, you will need to inform the emergency room doctor or nurse of your medications. I also recommend that patients enroll in the Medic Alert Program (1-800-736-3342); patients wear a bracelet or necklace that identifies their medical condition, treating doctor, and allergies, or provides other critical medical information. At the end of this chapter, I include a medication chart that I commonly use. I usually write the medications and dosing times in pencil so that they can be frequently updated. Many patients miniaturize this chart, and I have seen numerous variations that range from nothing more than a hand-scribbled note to a sophisticated computer printout by patients so inclined. The important message here, however, is always to carry with you a current list of all your medications, including not only your prescription medications but also all the nonprescription medications (minerals, vitamins, aspirin, cold remedies, and so on) that you might be taking.

TIPS ON TAKING YOUR MEDICINES

1. Know the name, dosage, actions, special instructions, and common side effects of all the medicines you are taking. Keep your medications handy. Bring them to all visits to your doctor's office.

2. Take your medicines as ordered. Even when you are feeling better, continue taking them on schedule. Never take more than has been prescribed, and do not stop taking them unless told to do so by your doctor.

3. It is preferable that you take your medicines at the same time each day to ensure a consistent level of the medicine in your bloodstream. If you have trouble figuring out a convenient schedule, ask for help. Sometimes, following the chart shown at the end of this chapter is helpful.

4. Keep your medicines in their original containers. Do not remove labels.

5. Ask your doctor before taking any over-the-counter medicines (including Dristan, Sudafed, Anacin, or any other cold pills or pain relievers, even aspirin).

6. Medicines can become outdated and therefore ineffective. If they are more than several months old, ask your pharmacist or doctor if they are still effective and safe.

7. Do not give your medicines to anyone, even if that person seems to have the same symptoms as you do.

8. It may take time for your body to adjust to a new medicine, and it may take time for the medicine to begin to work effectively. Sometimes, you may have mild side effects during this period. Discuss them with your doctor. Sometimes, another medicine can be prescribed. However, always report anything unusual when taking a new medication.

9. When a new medicine is prescribed, ask your pharmacist to give you only a one- or two-week supply until you are sure your body will tolerate it. (Your doctor may give you samples to see if you tolerate the new medication.) Call your doctor if you are running low on the samples to see if he or she wants you to continue with that medication.

10. Cost can be an important factor with medicines, since most prescribed drugs can be expensive. However, you cannot afford *not* to take them. Discuss this with your doctor. Perhaps less expensive medicines can be substituted. Also, ask your doctor about available indigent programs, if you have such a need.

11. Many times there are helpful warnings and instructions on prescription bottles. For example, these may remind you to take the medication with food or after a meal. Generally, you should heed these instructions. However, patients sometimes run into problems with the warnings on bottles of potassium supplements, which advise taking these "with plenty of water." Since that is generally not the best advice for most heart failure patients, be sure to check with your doctor for more specific instructions.

12. If you miss a dose of a medication, check with your doctor rather than take an extra dose. Doses of certain heart failure medications too close together can often do more harm than good. Try *not* to miss doses.

COMMON HEART FAILURE MEDICATIONS

In this section, I list several of the drugs that are commonly used in treating patients with heart failure. I first list the generic name for the drug, as well as some of the common brand names for it. Then I provide some general information about the drug, list the common dose range, and some of the common side effects. I then list some of the possible interactions.

Before I discuss each of the drug categories, I am going to remind you of what one of my senior residents told me when I was an intern. He said, "Any drug can do anything." Basically, what he meant was that since most drugs can potentially produce a wide range of actions and side effects, you should take it seriously when a patient reports an unusual effect from a medication. I have always done so, even when the textbooks don't report a certain reaction. Everyone reacts differently to medications. Frankly, it is quite surprising to me how many people really do tolerate the many medications we use for treating heart failure.

As I mentioned earlier, there are many good books available that detail all of the effects, side effects, and dosages of drugs (some even show pictures of the medications), and patients should refer to these. Almost everyone has access to a public library, which should contain one of the books that lists all the medications. For example, the *Physicians' Desk Reference (PDR)*, which is updated every year, lists all the information available on over 3,000 drugs. You can look any drug up in this book, either by its generic name or its brand name, and read a brief description of it, including some of the clinical pharmacology about the drug as well as its indications and usage. The *PDR* also lists contraindications, or reasons you should not take the drug; warnings, particularly regarding the use of drugs during pregnancy, important precautions, and adverse reactions that may occur. Commonly, there is also a section on interactions with other drugs and specific information on what to do in the event of an overdose, as well as information regarding the specific dosage and administration, although, many times, the drugs that are used for heart failure are used in dosages that may differ from those listed for other indications, such as high blood pressure. Finally, the *PDR* will give you information about how the medication is supplied, that is, in what form and dosage. There is even a pictorial guide so that you can match up your pills with the picture to make sure you are taking the correct pill and the right dosage.

When your doctor prescribes a new medication, frequently, he or she will give you a sample with a package insert that contains the same printed information that appears in the *PDR*. When you go to a pharmacy to pick up a new prescription, you may want to ask the pharmacist to give you a copy of the package insert, which will detail all of this information. Many pharmacies nowadays provide either computer printouts or standardized forms that describe a bit more about the medication the patient is taking, and because many pharmacies have all of a person's prescriptions on a computer, they can easily identify any potential interactions among the drugs that person is taking.

I think these are very positive moves, and I encourage most of my patients to refer to the *PDR* or a similar kind of text to learn more about their medications. At the same time, however, I also warn them that if they read about any drug they are afraid to take, that some faith has to be placed in their physician to prescribe the proper medication and the proper dosage best to treat their heart failure.

Recently I explored the health section of one of the on-line computer services that are becoming so popular. A subscriber can look up a drug and read information on its indications, how to take the medication, what to do about missed doses, and so on. However, I think it would be rather frightening for a patient to read about all the side effects that were listed without having a physician, nurse, or pharmacist there to add a comment or two about how often these side effects actually occur in their experience. I believe more and more people will probably get their drug information in this way as we expand our "communication superhighways," and I hope this process does not have a negative effect on doctor-patient relationships or on a patient's compliance with medications.

Digoxin

The common brand name for digoxin is Lanoxin.

General Information.   Digoxin is a medication that is commonly used to help the heart beat stronger and somewhat slower and more regularly. It is commonly used to control irregular heart rhythms, such as atrial fibrillation, but has also been shown to improve the heart's pumping function. Digitalis, an older preparation of this drug made directly from the foxglove plant, is rarely used today.

Common Dosages. Digoxin is used in a variety of dosages, ranging from 0.125 milligrams to 0.375 milligrams daily, and is usually taken as a single dose. However, digoxin is one of those medications for which the dosage is greatly dependent on many other conditions, such as age, kidney function, and other medications you are taking. Therefore, the dosage has to be adjusted carefully by your doctor and may even change as you take other medicines. Some patients may only take doses several times a week, rather than daily.

Common Side Effects. Digoxin is a medication that can have a fairly high incidence of side effects, primarily because of all the drug interactions and conditions that alter the level of digoxin in a patient's blood. Up to 30 percent of all hospitalized patients taking digoxin have some degree of toxicity from it. Most of the side effects, however, usually indicate that the patient has too much digoxin in his or her system. This is called digoxin toxicity. Loss of appetite and nausea can be very early side effects, indicating that there is too much digoxin in the blood. A patient may also have blurred vision or see a yellow halo around objects and lights, and may have serious, as well as nonserious, irregular heartbeats and excessive slowing of the pulse. Occasionally, digoxin causes some increase in and tenderness of the breast tissue in both men and women. The dosage of digoxin needs to be carefully monitored and adjusted in anyone who has an impairment in kidney function, a common condition in patients who have heart failure and in elderly patients. Impaired function can lead to increased digoxin in the blood.

One of the side effects that I have become more aware of with digoxin is its effect on sexual function. Overall, this is small but can be quite problematic to an individual patient. In one large study on male sexual dysfunction, digoxin seemed to be the culprit on many occasions. If you are worried that digoxin is causing this side effect in you, I would suggest you discuss this with your doctor.

Drug Interactions. When taking digoxin, patients need an adequate amount of potassium and magnesium in their blood. Many drugs can raise the level of digoxin in the blood, including quinidine, verapamil, and amiodarone (Cordarone). Also, certain antibiotics, such as erythromycin, may increase the absorption of digoxin. Even certain foods can interact with the absorption of this medication; eating oat bran at the same time you take your digoxin dose can alter absorption and give you a lower level of digoxin in the blood than expected. Certain antacids, on the other hand, can also lower the absorption.

Most problems with digoxin occur when there is too much of it in the blood. The following conditions can predispose a person to digoxin toxicity:

1. Kidney failure
2. Too little potassium, too little magnesium, or too much calcium
3. Severe heart disease (NYHA Class III or IV)
4. A recent heart attack
5. Advanced age
6. Thyroid disease, especially hypothyroidism (underactive thyroid)
7. Hypoxic states (not enough oxygen)
8. Multiple drug therapy (especially including quinidine or amiodarone)
9. Other heart problems, including preexisting electrical abnormalities of the heart (AV [atrioventricular] block)

Diuretics (Water Pills)

Diuretics are a general class of medications that help the body rid itself of extra fluid. There are various types of water pills that act on different portions of the kidney. The majority of patients end up taking one of what we call the "loop" diuretics, such as furosemide. (The loop is a special part of the kidney.) Table 8.1 lists some common diuretics, along with their brand names and usual dosages.

General Information. Through a variety of different actions in the kidney, diuretics help to rid the body of excess fluid. Some diuretics, such as spironolactone, triamterene, and amiloride, help retain potassium in the bloodstream, whereas others tend to cause loss of potassium in the urine. Because these drugs help get rid of fluid, they can cause light-headedness, fatigue, thirst, diarrhea, or constipation. Usually, the side effects are caused by the alteration of

TABLE 8.1 Common Diuretics

Common brand name	Generic name	Usual dosage
Aldactone	Spironolactone	25–100 mg/day
Bumex	Bumetanide	0.5–20 mg/day
Demadex	Torsemide	10–100 mg/day
Diuril	Chlorothiazide	50–100 mg/day
Dyrenium	Triamterene	100–300 mg/day
Edecrin	Ethacrynic acid	50–200 mg/day
Hygroton	Chlorthalidone	25–100 mg/day
Lasix	Furosemide	20–400 mg/day
Midamor	Amiloride	5–10 mg/day
Zaroxolyn	Metolazone	2.5–10 mg/day

levels of electrolytes or other chemicals within the body. For example, by lowering the potassium level too much, diuretics can precipitate irregular heartbeats, weakness, and even cardiac arrest. They also occasionally cause skin rashes and hives. Calcium loss from chronic use can lead to osteoporosis or bone weakening in some patients. Another possible side effect is an increase in the uric acid level, which can precipitate an episode of gout. The thiazides (chlorothiazide, chlorthalidone, hydrochlorothiazide) can alter the cholesterol level, and furosemide and ethacrynic acid can cause hearing damage.

Interactions. Many diuretics contain sulfa, and a person with a sulfa allergy can be highly sensitive to these drugs (ethacrynic acid, however, does *not* contain sulfa). Diuretics can also interact with a wide variety of the so-called nonsteroidal anti-inflammatory drugs, such as Indocin or Motrin (ibuprofen). They can also cause sensitivity to sunlight (this may be particularly true of triamterene).

Because these medications cause an increase in urination, patients, particularly at night, should therefore avoid taking a dose of a diuretic immediately before going to bed.

Angiotensin-Converting Enzyme Inhibitors (ACEIs)

There is a wide variety of ACEIs currently available. Commonly used ACEIs include captopril (brand name, Capoten), enalapril (Vasotec), quinapril (Accupril), and Iisinopril (Prinivil, Zestril). The doses of these drugs vary a great deal depending on a patient's ability to tolerate the drug and on underlying conditions, such as renal function and age. There seems to be wide variation among physicians not only in terms of the dose they prescribe but also in the regimen they suggest for taking these medications. There is still a question regarding whether higher or lower doses of the ACEIs are needed to treat heart failure adequately, and a clinical trial is currently under way to help answer that question. Therefore, with a drug like Capoten, for example, often some patients will take as little as 6.25 milligrams twice per day, whereas others may take up to 75 milligrams four times per day. Generally, I like my patients to take Capoten at least three or four times per day in the highest dose they can tolerate. The typical dosage with Vasotec ranges anywhere from 2.5 milligrams once per day to 10 milligrams twice per day; I generally recommend twice daily dosing in the largest dose tolerated. For example, the dosage used in several of the studies showing the effectiveness of Vasotec was 10 milligrams twice per day. When these drugs are used to treat high blood pressure, Capoten twice daily or Vasotec once daily is adequate, but for heart failure, more frequent doses are required. The usual dosage for lisinopril (Prinivil, Zestril) is 5 to 20 milligrams once per day.

General Information. ACEIs help open up the arteries of the body and are commonly used to treat high blood pressure and heart failure. We are discovering that these drugs actually do many other important things in the body. It is generally best to take these drugs on an empty stomach, before eating.

Common Side Effects. The most common side effects of ACEIs are cough, loss of taste, a drop in the blood pressure, and, occasionally, worsening of kidney function. These drugs can also cause sore throat, fever, skin rash, and what is known as *angioedema,* a condition in which a person's throat swells up, causing difficulty in breathing. On rare occasions they can also lower the white cell count, which makes fighting off infections more difficult. Since patients who are on diuretics may have more episodes of low blood pressure, sometimes diuretics are reduced a bit prior to starting an ACEI. Also, these drugs can help retain potassium in the bloodstream and therefore have to be used with caution in people who are already on potassium supplements or in those who are taking a diuretic that may retain additional potassium. Occasionally, some of the anti-inflammatory drugs, even aspirin, can increase the potential of an ACEI to worsen kidney function, and recently, it has been suggested that aspirin may in fact negate some of the effect of an ACEI. A large trial, however, found that this does not seem to be the case. It has also been found that patients taking lithium can have a much higher level of lithium in the blood when taking one of the ACEIs.

Beta-Blockers

See the discussion above for the important role beta-blockers play in the treatment of heart failure. In general, since they are so important we generally recommend a start low, go slow, but steady uptitration approach to these drugs.

General Information. Beta-blockers can slow the heart rate but also allow the heart to recover function and improve symptoms and survival.

Common Side Effects: I have already mentioned the early worsening including tiredness and fluid retention. Again, these occur less frequently than

TABLE 8.2 Beta-blockers

Common Brand Name	Generic name	Start dose	Usual dosage
Coreg	Carvedilol	3.125 mg twice/day	6.25–25 mg twice/day
Toprol XL	Metoprolol CR/XL	12.5–25 mg /day	200 mg /day
Zebeta	Bisoprolol	2.5 mg /day	7.5–10 mg /day

one would suspect and can usually be managed by an alert doctor-patient team. Also they can cause slow heart rates, or even degrees of heart block. (As a note, some doctors feel so strongly about the value of these drugs that if heart block occurs or the heart rate gets too slow a pacemaker will be considered just to allow patients to receive these drugs.) Other side effects include dizziness, weight gain, nausea, and headache.

Interactions.   Using beta-blockers can interact with other drugs that may slow the heart rate such as digoxin or amiodarone. They can mask a response patients who are diabetics get if their blood sugar gets too low. This was once thought to be a reason not to use these drugs in diabetics but it now seems clear that diabetics value from these drugs as well.

Nitroglycerin

There are many ways in which nitroglycerin can be introduced into the bloodstream. There are pills that are either placed under the tongue or swallowed, as well as patches and creams that are absorbed through the skin. See Table 8.3 for the common brand name and usual dosages.

General Information.   Nitroglycerin is used to help dilate the veins and arteries and to improve blood flow to the heart; it may also improve blood flow through the lungs.

Common Dosages.   The dosages and administration patterns vary so much with the various nitroglycerin medications that you should consult your physician for further information. In general, these drugs are underdosed, in my opinion, because of concern about low blood pressure.

Common Side Effects.   Common side effects with nitroglycerin include flushing of the face and neck and headache, which occur usually shortly after taking the medication. Nitroglycerin can also cause skin rashes, a fast heart rate,

TABLE 8.3 Nitroglycerin

Common brand name	Generic name	Usual dosage
Imdur	Isosorbide mononitrate	30–120 mg once/day
Ismo	Isosorbide mononitrate	10–40 mg twice/day
Isordil tablets or capsules	Isosorbide dinitrate	10–40 mg 3 or 4 times/day
Nitro-Dur and Transderm-Nitro	Nitroglycerin patches	0.2–0.6 mg/hour

and dizziness or light-headedness, especially when the patient gets up from a seated position. Frequently, the headaches can be minimized by taking Tylenol prior to taking the medication. Nitroglycerin patches can cause irritation to the skin, which can be minimized by rotating the patch from site to site. Doctors used to recommend that the patches be worn an entire day at a time, but doctors now commonly suggest that they be removed for at least eight hours during the day to maximize their effectiveness and avoid what is called nitrate tolerance. This is especially true in patients using these drugs to treat *angina pectoris* (chest pain).

Interactions. Because nitroglycerin can lower blood pressure and open up the arteries, it certainly can worsen or accentuate the feeling of light-headedness that is produced by other medicines that also lower blood pressure, such as diuretics, ACEIs, and other vasodilators.

Other Vasodilators

There are other drugs besides the ACEIs—for example, hydralazine (a common brand name is Apresoline)—that open up the arteries. In fact, some of them have been used longer than the ACEIs. I am going to mention two classes of these drugs—direct vasodilators, such as hydralazine, and calcium channel blockers, such as diltiazem or nifedipine—because they are still commonly used for people who cannot tolerate the ACEIs; sometimes they are even used in addition to the ACEIs.

General Information. Vasodilators act directly on the arteries to increase their diameter and thereby decrease the resistance that the failing heart has to pump against. In fact, it was the combination of this medication (hydralazine) and isosorbide dinitrate that was one of the first combinations shown to lower the mortality rate of patients who had heart failure.

Common Dosages. The usual dosage of hydralazine is 10 to 75 milligrams three to four times per day, but, as is true of so many other medicines we have discussed, there is a wide range of dosing and frequency in the clinical use of this drug. It is my practice to generally maximize the dose and have patients take this drug four times a day. That was the regimen used in the trial that showed hydralazine to be so successful; until there is evidence otherwise, I generally try to duplicate the doses of drugs that were shown in studies to be useful. There are, however, many clinical situations in which lower doses of hydralazine are in fact used.

Common Side Effects. As you would expect with any drug that opens up the arteries, headache and low blood pressure—perhaps even a sudden drop in blood pressure—can occur. Hydralazine has some particular side effects, including a drug-related fever, skin rash, and, very frequently, a laboratory abnormality called a "positive antinuclear antibodies," which can indicate a lupuslike syndrome. (Systemic lupus erythematosus is a disease that can cause joint pain, skin rashes, and damage to the kidneys and many other organs.) Hydralazine can also cause headache, loss of appetite, nausea and vomiting, diarrhea, and even an - increased amount of chest pain in some patients.

Drug Interactions. Hydralazine may interact with any other drug that has some effect on blood pressure, and this drug should be used with extreme caution in patients receiving certain forms of antidepressants. When hydralazine is taken with food, there are higher levels of the drug in the blood; therefore, lower doses may be used.

Calcium Channel Blockers

Since calcium channel blockers also cause opening up of the arteries and veins, they are anticipated to have some use in treating heart failure. However, some of the older forms of these drugs also have the effect of making the heart muscle weaker and, therefore, are really of limited use in treating patients with heart failure. There are new calcium channel blockers that are being developed; in fact, clinical trials with at least a couple of them are now being conducted specifically in patients who have heart failure. In general, however, we rarely use these medications to treat heart failure without specific reasons.

Table 8.4 lists a few of the many calcium channel blockers. Although the jury is still out on the general usefulness of these drugs in treating heart failure, there are certain forms of heart failure, such as hypertrophic cardiomyopathy, for which these drugs are the mainstay of therapy. I suggest that you discuss these drugs with your doctor to see if they are useful for your particular form of heart failure.

As would be expected, hypotension is a common adverse effect with this group of drugs. They also can produce a rapid heartbeat and a sensation of palpitations along with flushing, headaches, and, commonly, leg edema that is not related to the degree of heart failure. Since they can also alter the electrical system of the heart to varying degrees and cause heart block (impaired electrical conduction between the upper and lower chambers of the heart), these drugs have to be used carefully with other drugs that have this effect, such as beta-blockers or digoxin.

TABLE 8.4 Common Calcium Channel Blockers

Common brand name	Generic name	Usual dosage
Calan	Verapamil	120–360 mg/day
Cardene	Nicardipine	60–120 mg/day
Cardizem or Dilacor XR	Diltiazem	90–240 mg/day
Norvasc	Amlodipine	5–20 mg/day
Plendil	Felodipine	5–10 mg/day
Procardia	Nifedipine	30–60 mg/day

Constipation, exacerbated by other heart failure medications and by the fluid restriction imposed on heart failure patients, is a common side effect with many calcium channel blockers and is the reason often cited by patients for drug intolerance.

Coumadin

Another drug commonly used in patients with heart failure is the medication known as warfarin sodium, commonly known by the brand name Coumadin. This drug is a potent medication that works as an anticoagulant, or blood thinner. Drugs of this type are used in patients with heart failure either to prevent the formation of blood clots in the heart to prevent the *embolization,* or breaking loose, of blood clots that may already be present in the heart. When a person has atrial fibrillation, the upper chambers of the heart are not beating on a regular basis, a condition that can result in *blood stasis,* or slowing of the current of circulating blood. Blood that is not being ejected from the upper chambers in a normal fashion can tend to clot, or coagulate. When a *thrombus,* or blood clot, forms, there is the risk that a microscopic portion of it might break off, go elsewhere in the body—to the brain, kidney, lung, even the intestine—and cause serious medical problems.

Blood clotting is also a problem when the heart muscle is weak—generally, with an ejection fraction of less than 25 percent, blood clots can form within the left ventricle. And since blood clots frequently form inside the heart muscle after large heart attacks, anticoagulants are used to prevent additional clots from forming and to allow the body to put a thin coating of tissue around the existing blood clots so that embolization is prevented.

Regardless of the reason for using a blood thinner, patients need to be aware that this medicine works by blocking the synthesis of some of the factors that normally allow the blood to clot. Most of these are factors dependent on vitamin K, and, in fact, changes in the diet either to increase or decrease the intake of foods rich in vitamin K can significantly alter the effectiveness of the blood thinner. Therefore, the patient should try to keep his or her intake of foods rich in vitamin K constant, if at all possible, when taking Coumadin. There are also various medications that interact with Coumadin to make it either more or less effective; such medications therefore expose the patient either to bleeding, if the anticoagulation capability becomes too extreme, or to additional risk of blood clotting. A great many substances can increase the activity of Coumadin and therefore increase the risk of bleeding, including alcohol, allopurinol, aspirin, amiodarone (Cordarone), many antibiotics, some diuretics, ibuprofen (Motrin), indomethacin (Indocin), naproxen (Naprosyn), quinidine, and thyroid medications. Medications that can decrease the activity of Coumadin and therefore increase the risk of blood clotting include antacids, antihistamines, many sleeping pills, oral contraceptives, and vitamin C.

Because of the narrow range of clotting ability in which the blood must be maintained, patients taking Coumdin are asked to have their blood checked frequently to make sure that it is clotting to the right degree. This is determined by measuring prothrombin time, better known as "pro time," or PT. Prothrombin is converted to thrombin in the body, which helps form blood clots. This simple test can be done at any laboratory by sampling blood either from a vein or from a finger prick. The pro time may be reported as the number of seconds it takes for the blood to clot compared to a normal control; it is now more commonly being reported as an International Normalized Ratio, or INR.

Coumadin therapy can be very important for patients with heart failure, damaged heart valves, or irregular heartbeats, but close followup by the physician and frequent checks on adequate anticoagulation are necessary. This certainly is one situation where patients should discuss any planned surgery—no matter how minor—with the doctor who manages their heart failure, and there must always be a single doctor in charge of management of Coumadin therapy. Patients taking Coumadin should also discuss with that doctor any additional medication another doctor may prescribe, including any over-the-counter medication.

I think in the next few years we will have a better understanding as to whether chronic use of warfarin benefits patients with heart failure. It is possible that aspirin alone for most patients may be most beneficial in terms of clot prevention. You should also ask about a Coumadin clinic which might help your doctor better monitor your dose and be alert for side effects.

Potassium Supplements

Potassium supplements are often prescribed for patients taking diuretics. As I mentioned earlier, when increased urine is passed through the kidney, potassium, along with other electrolytes, is frequently excreted in increased amounts as well. On the basis of an analysis of the potassium level in your blood, and in consideration of the other medications you might be taking that may have any effect on either retaining or losing potassium, your doctor may recommend that you take a potassium supplement. A normal amount of potassium is critical for the day-to-day functioning of your body. There are an enormous number of potassium products available on the market, and your physician will try to find a product that will work for you and that is most convenient for you. These products come in tablet, liquid, and powder form, and most patients have their preference. Many patients with heart failure end up taking extremely large doses of potassium because of the large doses of diuretics they are on; to reduce the number of potassium pills or the amount of liquid a patient must consume, a physician might decide at some point to prescribe an additional medicine that helps retain potassium. These specifics should be discussed directly with your doctor. There are also problems that can develop with too much potassium; these typically occur in patients who had kidney malfunction or are taking drugs that help retain potassium, such as spironolactone or even the ACEIs, such as captopril or enalapril. Potassium can be irritating to the stomach and intestinal tract. Generally, heart failure patients take these medications at meals with some fluid, although, because of the fluid restriction, most of these patients are not on as much fluid as pharmacists usually recommend.

Lately, I have been asked about patients taking potassium supplements that are available at health food stores. Although the potassium salt is acceptable, the problem is that most of these over-the-counter preparations have low concentrations. The average heart failure patient takes 20 milliequivalents of potassium twice per day, the equivalent of 1,500 milligrams of potassium twice per day, and most prescription potassium tablets or liquids come in doses between 600 and 1,500 milligrams per tablet or spoonful. The common health food store preparations I have seen contain somewhere between 50 and 90 milligrams, so a patient would end up taking many of these potassium pills to get the same effect. Unless you have discussed this with your doctor and it has been determined that the potassium supplement you find in the health food store can adequately replace your potassium losses, this would not be a wise gamble.

One of the common effects of a low potassium level is the muscle cramps that generally occur in the legs, feet, or even the hands. It is important to know that a variety of other electrolyte imbalances, such as low calcium, low magnesium, or low sodium, can also cause these cramps, as can certain medications, including nifedipine (Procardia), terbutaline (Brethine), cimetidine (Tagamet), and lithium. Actually, in most cases, the cause is usually not found. Leg cramps that occur at night are particularly disturbing; they may awaken the person from sleep and may last from several minutes to several hours. They occur more frequently as a person ages, and it has been estimated that up to 70 percent of people over the age of fifty have some form of nocturnal leg cramps. However, for patients with heart failure who are taking large doses of diuretics and potassium, I always think it is worthwhile to check the potassium level when the patient reports such cramps. When the cramps continue despite normal levels of electrolytes, then other avenues can be pursued. Doctors commonly prescribe quinine pills; I often suggest that patients take small sips of quinine water or tonic water. A recent study comparing quinine to vitamin E showed that quinine was the only effective treatment. There are other drugs available, but often, some simple exercises that a doctor can recommend may be all that's needed for most cases of leg cramps. The important point here is that since muscle cramps may be a sign that potassium is low, you should be alert to them and report any occurrence to your doctor.

Patient: _____

Medications	6 AM	7 AM	8 AM	9 AM	10 AM	11 AM	12 Nn	1 PM	2 PM	3 PM	4 PM	5 PM	6 PM	7 PM	8 PM	9 PM	10 PM	11 PM	12 Md	1 AM	2 AM	3 AM	4 AM	5 AM

FIGURE 8.1 Heart failure medication schedule

9

Heart Transplantation

For many years of my professional life, I watched and worked with the miracle of heart transplantation. For many patients with very advanced heart failure, this operation is lifesaving and restores them to health for quite some time. But I would be lying to readers if I were to say that transplantation is a "cure" for heart failure. I believe the more balanced view is to say that it is a compromise, exchanging one set of problems (those of heart failure) with another set of problems (those of heart transplantation).

To be able to talk about heart transplantation as an everyday event, when not so long ago this phenomenon was considered to be in the realm of science fiction, is truly remarkable. However, after years of research and hard work, primarily by the pioneers of heart transplantation at Stanford University, heart transplants are in fact an everyday occurrence here in the United States and worldwide. From my years of serving as a heart transplant cardiologist, I have great respect for this procedure that can transform a critically ill heart failure patient into someone who has enormous vigor and stamina. However, there remain many caveats for most patients with heart failure, and I want to review some of these briefly.

The first thing to consider are the numbers, which play an important role in understanding how transplantation fits into the treatment picture for heart failure. Despite the major advances that have been made in heart transplantation, the cold, hard fact is that there are a limited number of donor organs. There are many reasons for this, but it seems that we have reached a plateau, with approximately 3,000 heart transplants being done annually worldwide and probably about 2,000 of those being done in the United States. In fact, according to the most recent official report of the registry of the International Society for Heart and Lung Transplantation, the total number of transplants performed worldwide dipped to less than 3,100 in 1996, well below the more than 20,000 to 30,000 recipients that could meet criteria and use a heart. What that means, in effect, is that the availability of donor organs is far less than the need for them. Many attempts have been made to educate the public in general about the desperate need for donor organs, but there has been little success. Unfortunately, there is a great deal of mythologizing about heart transplantation, and this has kept families from allowing their loved ones to become organ donors. The tabloid stories of organs sold on a "black market" do nothing but inhibit much-needed organ donation. Nonetheless, even if we were to double, triple, or even quadruple the number of organ donors, it would barely touch the problem for the millions of patients who have advanced heart failure.

The major question, then, is who should be selected to receive a heart transplant? The criteria have certainly changed since heart transplantation first began in the early 1960s and have even changed within the past decade. By and large, the person who needs a heart transplant is someone who has end-stage heart disease and is no longer amenable to medical or other surgical treatments. Obviously, however, since the wait can be quite long for a donor organ, we no longer want to select patients who are so far advanced that his or her survival is measured in days, weeks, or even months. Because of the high demand for donor organs, people may wait for a heart transplant for many months or even well beyond a year, without getting the call to receive their new heart. That leaves it up to the referring doctor to decide when the patient should be referred. I generally encourage referrals to heart transplant centers sooner rather than later. If the referral is made at too late a stage in the disease process, the patient often will not survive to get the heart transplant. When the referral is made early, the patient benefits, because, frequently, the staff at a heart transplant center is also experienced in caring for heart failure patients and can look at other options besides transplantation or use other treatments while the patient waits for the transplant.

Still another trend in transplantation that has occurred over the past several years has been the use of artificial devices, usually left ventricular assist devices for patients waiting to receive a new heart. Since donor shortages remain and potential recipients keep increasing, there is an enormous imbalance in the supply-demand ratio. Because of this, many ill patients go through several stages after being placed on a heart transplant list. These stages can vary in length but usually span months to years and include

- The patient waits at home, taking just oral medicines.
- The patient is admitted to the hospital because of worsening, is placed on continuous intravenous medicines to help the heart, and remains in an intensive care unit.

- The patient experiences further deterioration and the surgical placement of a mechanical device to support the heart. With some of these devices, a patient can go home, but the usual scenario is that the patient is so weak and debilitated that he or she usually remains in the hospital or initially goes to a center for rehabilitation. If successful, we feel these devices allow greater mobility and prevent some of the further deterioration of the other organs and muscles. The risk of infection always exists when a device is hooked up via an external drive line.
- Transplantation occurs more frequently than not, but not without a tremendous amount of coordinated work, dedication, and expense to get a patient to this point. The economics of it all are beyond the scope of this book, but suffice it to say that it is a huge problem. Daily, I do battle with insurers who are unwilling to understand the changing face of transplantation—that, increasingly, a decision to transplant is also in the best interest of the patient, a decision to place and maintain a device for support while awaiting a new heart.

The kinds of devices include left ventricular assist devices, which are pumps of various designs that simply take over the work of the main pumping chamber, the left ventricle. Until now, these have required large battery packs connected to a "drive line" through the skin. Newer models have smaller battery packs, and, in fact, many patients who get these new devices can work, exercise, and so on, mostly without noticing that they are on these devices. Newer devices will eliminate the need for the external drive line, with the energy transfer taking place through the skin. This will decrease the risks of infection. Even newer devices will be totally implantable with internal energy sources. Increasingly, as we gain more experience, we find that sometimes the effectiveness of the assist device allows some recovery of the patient's heart, and we occasionally think of removing the device. This trend toward "bridge to recovery" is becoming more popular.

For patients whose right ventricle is still functioning, then the LVAD (left ventricular assist device) is usually all they need. However for some patients with a failing right ventricle as well, we need to consider a total artificial heart. I have been fortunate to continue to work with these devices and find them lifesaving. The power supply is a large, bulky one, and so we truly try to get a new donor heart as soon as possible. For these patients, because their original heart is totally removed to put in the device, there is no hope for a bridge to recovery.

Besides a severely damaged heart, there are other criteria that determine who can become a heart transplant recipient. A person should have no other organs that are failing. In other words, although the heart may be severely affected, a good candidate for transplantation has kidneys, lungs, liver, and so on in good working order, thus allowing for a good recovery after the heart transplant and limiting future complications. Additionally, there should not be any serious psychological or social problems, since the burden of waiting for and then receiving a new heart, along with the psychological effects of the immunosuppressive medication, can worsen any existing psychological problem the patient may have. Conditions such as drug or alcohol abuse, an unstable family situation, or a family lacking strong supports are frequently reasons to exclude someone as a possible heart transplant recipient. Another complicating problem can be a serious illness that affects the body as a whole, such as lupus erythematosus or insulin-requiring diabetes.

The question of age is a common one: Who is too old to receive a heart transplant? One of the interesting things that we have learned over the past decade is that the older patients do not do any worse than younger patients when it comes to receiving a heart transplant. Indeed, there is some evidence that suggests that the older person with the more quiescent immune system fares even better than the younger patient. Therefore, it is not unusual to see patients even well into their sixties being considered for heart transplantation.

To summarize, the ideal heart transplantation candidate is someone who has very advanced heart failure with a reasonable one-year life expectancy, who does not have any other major illness or any other organ that is severely affected, and who has a strong psychological and social support system. However, because of the limited number of donor organs available, the candidate must often be one who has tried and failed other conventional and even experimental treatment programs.

With that in mind, I consider what might be involved should a patient require a heart transplant evaluation. Unfortunately, one of the primary considerations is the form of insurance coverage a patient has. Not all insurance policies will cover transplant services, and patients often discover these limitations too late. Usually, when a doctor refers a patient to a heart transplant center, the center will screen the patient's insurance coverage prior to beginning any further evaluation. After the first hurdle is cleared in terms of assuring insurance coverage or clarifying the financial arrangements, there is usually an extensive review of the testing that has already been performed as a preliminary screen to make sure that the person is indeed a reasonable candidate. Then the patient is commonly admitted to the heart transplant center for a short evaluation, which often includes repeating some of the tests that were done in the past, such as an echocardiogram, a MUGA test, and blood tests. Frequently, the patient and the family meet with a social worker, a psychologist or psychiatrist, or both to determine the extent of support that will be available and the potential for psychological problems. Actually, I think most patients find this part of the evaluation a relief, for it helps to bring to the forefront some of the anxieties that are present in anyone who has suffered from heart failure for many years.

Since patients often have to wait so long for a heart to become available, as I mentioned earlier, the process of actually trying to pick the optimal timing for a heart transplant and to decide which patients can wait longer for a transplant and which cannot is a critical part of the transplant evaluation. Earlier, I talked about the cardiopulmonary exercise (CPX) test and the important information it gives us in evaluating patients with heart failure and in predicting long-term survival (see Chapter 3). Heart transplant centers use this technique to help them decide who needs a heart transplant and when. Recent studies have shown that patients who do well on the CPX test can be reasonably managed on medical treatments alone and may in fact not need a heart transplant. On the other hand, a poor performance would suggest the need for heart transplantation earlier rather than later.

One of the tests that is frequently repeated at a heart transplant center is the placement of a Swan-Ganz catheter to measure the pressures within the heart and lungs. This test not only determines the absolute pressures but also assesses the degree to which the high pressures in the lungs and heart can be reversed. This, of course, is a critically important determination to make. If a patient has very high pressures in the lungs that cannot be reversed simply by putting in a new heart or pump, the new heart will be damaged by the high pressures almost immediately. Recognizing this fact was instrumental in helping us overcome some of the early disasters in heart transplantation. There are a variety of medicines that can be used to test whether the pressures in a patient's lungs can be lowered and to predict how the patient might do after the damaged heart is replaced with a new one. If the pressure in the lungs cannot be suitably lowered, the transplant doctors begin to think of alternative strategies for the patient, including implanting a donor heart that is larger than normal or even transplanting both a new heart and lungs. Occasionally, it may mean declaring the patient to be unsuitable for transplantation.

At the end of the transplant evaluation, a judgment is made as to whether the patient is a candidate for a transplant at that time or judgment will be deferred. If the patient does become a transplant candidate and is put on an active waiting list, a period of great stress and emotional turmoil then begins. As one of my patients told me years ago, "This is really an awkward feeling, because you are waiting to live while you are waiting for another person to die." Such thoughts and feelings, as well as the constraints imposed on the patient's lifestyle by the heart failure, make this a very stressful time for patient and family alike.

I think it is important to say a few words about organ donors. As you would expect, organ donors are usually young people who have suffered some kind of injury and cannot be kept alive without artificial means, but whose organs are undamaged. Typically, this is a young person who has been in a motor vehicle accident and has suffered brain death, but whose other organs are functioning normally. Frequently, multiple organs, including kidneys, liver, heart, and lungs, are donated. A great deal of effort has gone into educating medical centers in this country on how to identify and take care of a potential organ donor, so that organs that can be used for life in other patients are salvaged and preserved.

Because of the short supply of organs for transplantation, some of the early stringent criteria applied to organ donors are now obsolete. I remember when we would automatically turn down a potential heart donor over the age of thirty-five. Now, with the ability to assess a donor's heart function with echoes and with angiograms to look at the arteries to make sure they are normal, older organ donors are being carefully considered. Interestingly, a friend of mine in California has attempted a program of matching older, less optimal recipients with less suitable donors, a "B" list, so to speak. These are candidates who would otherwise not be eligible for a donor heart; this system exists to make sure that these recipients don't consume the best available donors. In fact, the early results of this program have been quite acceptable and have taught us a lot about donor selection.

Although I said earlier that the number of organ donors could never keep pace with the number of potential recipients, I think we should nevertheless continue to increase awareness of the need for organ donors. I have seen the families of many patients become interested in being organ donors themselves and place organ donation stickers on their driver's license during the period of time when their loved one was waiting for a heart transplant. I think the decision to become an organ donor is best done with forethought, and I believe the topic of organ donation should be discussed among families, with members making their wishes known, at a time when the family is not in crisis. I do not think I can recall a single instance where an organ donor's family regretted having donated organs to a needy individual.

Other questions that are often asked about heart transplantation involve some of the hard data, including the overall survival statistics and what life is like after a heart transplant. I think many of these issues are best discussed with the staff of individual transplant centers, but I'd like to give some brief outlines to clear up any of the myths surrounding heart transplantation. The overall one-year survival rate for patients undergoing routine heart transplantation is currently somewhere between 80 and 90 percent. Even five years after transplantation, more than 70 percent of the patients remain alive. This is a remarkable contrast to the survival statistics gathered when heart transplantation was in its infancy in the early 1960s. Various factors are responsible for this marked improvement, especially our ability to biopsy the heart and look for rejection and the development of better immunosuppressive drugs, particularly cyclosporine. It was really the introduction of this drug that made heart transplantation a procedure that could be done in many medical centers rather than in just a few specialized ones. Another major advance has been the development of sophisticated heart transplant teams who are aware of all the problems a patient may have in both the pre- and the posttransplant period.

A heart biopsy remains the best way to look for evidence of rejection of the heart. Biopsies are usually done within the first several months after transplantation and are continued at less frequent intervals, if the patient's condition warrants, for the entire life of the patient. There is also frequent monitoring of immunosuppressive drug levels, and transplant cardiologists are always on the lookout for the development of a special kind of rejection that causes blocking of the arteries, which could lead to a heart attack or even sudden death. As you may know, the new heart is placed into the chest cavity without any nerves attacked to the patient; therefore, any difficulty the heart may have may go undetected because of the person's inability to feel pain. The patient with a heart transplant lives a scrutinized life, but virtually none of the transplant patients I know would trade this life for their former one of advanced heart failure.

There are various other problems that go with heart transplantation, including high blood pressure, excess hair growth, elevation of the blood lipids, and the omnipresent risk of serious infection. Nonetheless, I think patients feel that the heart transplant is their last chance for survival, and the majority of patients enjoy a great deal of symptomatic relief. I think everyone has seen a picture of the heart transplant softball teams or picnics that take place throughout this country. It is certainly rewarding to see very sick people transformed into healthy ones. We can only be hopeful that further advances not only in transplanting donor hearts but also in finding better, safer ways for detecting rejection of the heart and for immunosuppressing the patient will be made in the decades ahead.

Many of the heart transplant programs have strong support groups not only for patients who have already had their transplant but also for those who are waiting for a transplant. Perhaps a support group is a good place for the heart failure patient considering transplantation to start; the group can give such an individual a patient's perspective on the pleasures and problems of heart transplantation.

Finally, I think one question that is not discussed but must certainly be on the mind of every patient who waits for and gets a new heart is "How long is this going to last?" We'd like to say the transplanted heart is just as good as a new heart, but that's simply not true. Because of the immunosuppression and the ongoing levels of rejection, the transplanted heart lasts a shorter period of time. Again, the International Society of Heart and Lung Transplantation statistics tell us the "half-life" for transplantation is about eight years, which means that about 50 percent of patients will die within eight years after a transplant. In my experience, even this number is unusual, and I'd like to say that I've seen lots of heart transplant programs filled with sixteen-year and beyond survivors. That is not the case. Fortunately, I think the way most heart transplant recipients deal with this is by focusing on the positives—the greatness of their gift, enjoying their good health, and saying, "I'm going to break the records."

The real hope is that soon, better options, beyond transplantation, will be available for more patients with advanced heart failure, and perhaps there will even be devices that will allow failed transplant patients to look beyond an otherwise certain grimness. These options will be discussed in the chapters that follow.

10

Experimental Approaches for Treating Heart Failure:
What Clinical Trials Are All About

Getting the Latest Advances Today

"The experiment of yesterday is the science of today and the dogma of tomorrow." No one famous made this statement—I made it up because it reflects what I believe is the truth about investigational treatments. What is experimental today will be what is used routinely tomorrow, that is, if it is proven to work and be safe! That is the purpose of doing the clinical trials or research.

That is why when I saw the recent cover of a popular magazine discussing clinical trials as the creation of human guinea pigs I was deeply saddened. Yes, there has been an increased awareness of some of the "scandals" that have taken place at some of the nation's major research institutions. But what is behind the scenes on these is that most of the "scandal" was some improper or sloppy paperwork. The most important facts in my mind are these:

- Patients in clinical trials get an opportunity to get the proven therapies of tomorrow, today.
- Patients in clinical trials receive close observation and superb treatment.
- The overwhelming majority of investigators and research nurses are ethical people who only want to help their patients.
- There is enormous scrutiny by review boards and trial sponsors to make sure that the best and safest care is being delivered to patients in the trials.

Currently there are several areas where I know in my heart that the investigational therapies being tried are working and yet it may be another two to five years before I can offer those treatments to the rest of my patients who are not eligible for the trials.

With almost every patient I see with heart failure, I end up discussing some of the experimental approaches for treatment at some point. I don't always do it at the first visit because, let's face it, the terms *experimental* and *investigational* conjure up the concept of a mad doctor in his lab doing work on guinea pigs. Because at some point you may be asked to consider some of these experimental approaches, I want to give you some of my strong opinions about what an experimental approach really is and how you should consider it.

First of all, you should remember that many of the drugs we are now using as conventional therapy went through periods of testing when they, in fact, were the new investigational drug. Take the example of the angiotensin-converting enzyme inhibitors (ACEIs), such as captopril or enalapril, which are now part of the core conventional treatment we use in so many patients with heart failure. It was only about a decade ago that these drugs were experimental. During my residency training, I remember quite clearly admitting patients to the hospital who were going to receive the drug captopril as an experimental agent. We took many precautions: We measured patients' blood pressure, ran blood chemistries and urine analyses, and examined patients closely each day, checking them in sitting and standing positions. Now, these drugs require a minimum of follow-up testing and are given out routinely by doctors all across the country. The ease with which we now use these drugs is the result of the many hours and long years of hard work that physicians and scientists devoted to their development. However, it is also due in great part to the many thousands of patients who participated in clinical trials using these drugs. I think those patients would agree that they benefited from a drug, established decades later as quite useful, much sooner than would otherwise have been possible.

When I have patients who are reluctant to participate in a clinical trial because they fear they are going to be treated as a guinea pig or have concerns about the effect of the drug, I (or one of my experienced nurses) usually tell them that, in my opinion, patients who enter clinical trials get even better care than those who do not. Not only do they get the frequent examinations and tests that are mandated by the treatment protocol, but also the amount of care and checkup they receive usually goes way beyond what is required by the sponsoring agency. There is always some complaint in the United States about a drug not being released at a fast enough rate or not being available here, although it is available in Europe, but I think, on the whole, that Americans are fortunate to have fair and compassionate rules regulating the development, testing, and introduction of new drugs.

If you are invited to participate in a clinical trial, you may want to ask some of the following key questions when discussing the investigational treatment with a physician or nurse. (You should know that before any human trials begin, there will have been extensive animal testing to delineate dosing and side effects.) First of all, you should know whether the study you are asked to participate in is a Phase II, a Phase III, or even a Phase IV trial. The differences have to do with the stage of development the drug is in, the number of people who have been exposed to it, and the questions that are being asked. Usually, Phase II trials involve the early development of the drug in human beings; they may, for example, be conducted to determine what the proper dosage should be. These trials are usually small, very well controlled, and of short duration.

A Phase III trial is usually broader, and the dosage has been well defined. The sponsoring agency is looking at the overall effectiveness of the drug as well as at any side effects that may not have been apparent in the past. It may also be looking at the overall efficacy and safety of the drug over a longer period of time.

A Phase IV trial involves a drug that is already on the market. The sponsor may now be looking at such issues as the efficacy of using the drug once per day rather than in a multiple-dose regimen, or may be comparing the drug to another one that is also already on the market.

With Phase II and Phase III drug trials, patients get the added benefit of receiving a drug long before it is approved. The Phase IV drug trial only asks patients to help answer a question about an already-approved drug; there is no benefit in terms of getting a truly experimental agent earlier than would otherwise be possible.

You should be aware that many drug trials are placebo controlled, which means that a certain percentage of the patients in a trial, frequently half, will get a *placebo,* or inert substance, and not the new drug in question. This is one of the main ways to determine if a new drug does what it is supposed to do. If, for example, the patients who got Drug *X* get much better, whereas those who got the placebo get much worse, then it is clear that Drug *X* is a good drug. However, the opposite can be true: There can be negative effects in the patients who got the drug as compared to those who got the placebo. These negative effects can be poor tolerance of the drug or even increased mortality. Commonly, in addition to being placebo controlled, drug trials are "double blind," which means that neither patients nor their doctors know who is getting the real drug and who is getting the placebo. There can also be a crossover; that is, for a period of time, the patient gets the real drug and then later crosses over to a period of placebo, or vice versa. Again, usually, neither the patient nor the doctor knows which substance, the drug or the placebo, is being given. A *randomized* study means that the sponsoring agency will determine which patients receive which substance and in what order; this is done to avoid any bias the doctor may have toward giving the real drug to the sicker patients and the placebo to the healthier ones.

Heart failure drug trials are usually looking for one of several effects or for a combination of effects. An effect can be an increase in survival rate, an increase in exercise tolerance, or, better yet, an improvement in the CPX test result or peak oxygen consumption. An effect can also be a decrease in the number of extra heartbeats, an improvement in the ejection fraction, or an overall improvement or amelioration of symptoms. Surprisingly, only recently have questionnaires been developed to measure a patient's quality of life, and that improvement in quality of life has been considered an important end point in a clinical trial.

Once a clinical trial is mentioned to you, you will usually be given written as well as other information regarding the purpose of the trial, its objectives, your exact risks and benefits, and your level of participation. You should study the written material carefully, but remember that you can pose any questions you may have directly to your doctors and nurses, who are the investigators for the trial. Doctors try to match their objectives and commitments for investigating a drug with their responsibilities in meeting their patients' needs. For example, I try to get patients who I think are on rather tenuous ground and with whom I'd like to try a new treatment into a treatment trial that is a Phase II or even a Phase III clinical trial of short duration, so that they are not committed to a trial that may go on for two or three years. That does not mean that if there should be a problem or a patient needs other treatment, he or she cannot get out of the trial; almost all trials have some fail-safe mechanism, so that the patient can exit the trial at any point. A good match should be attempted between a patient's clinical needs and the nature of the available trials.

Another issue that should not be overlooked is that in many clinical trials, there is financial support for much, if not all, of the testing to be done; often, patients are unlikely to incur any charge. Again, the physician investigator should try to match the patient's needs with the requirements of the trial. For example, for most patients, it is important to have a recent measurement of the pressures within the heart and lungs. This usually requires a brief hospital admission, but, as we all know, even a brief hospital admission can be expensive with today's hospital costs. Therefore, I will frequently match patients who are in need of such a measurement with an ongoing trial that will allow them to come into the hospital and get such a measurement without charge. Usually, as part of the trial, the measurements are made to investigate the effects of one or another drug on the pressures within the heart and lungs. Knowing these measurements is often of great benefit to me in planning treatment for the patient, and, in fact, a patient's participation in such a trial usually helps to determine whether a drug is potentially useful for treating his or her heart failure.

I think the key point here is that although clinical trials, investigational agents, and experimental drugs all sound very much like science fiction, they are actually an everyday part of medical care in this country. By and large, they represent an opportunity for your doctor to give you a new treatment for your heart failure that may not be available to the general public for many years to come. With the safety and monitoring requirements of federal and local agencies, these trials are conducted in a safe and efficient way. Although I mentioned earlier that patients are frequently reluctant to enter clinical trials, I think the more common situation is the reverse. Some patients are so eager to get into clinical trials, because there may be something new, something bigger and better, available for them, that they are ready to rush into the trials without understanding all the potential risks and benefits. Here is an example. Recently, there was quite a bit of publicity surrounding the early release of a drug that was still undergoing some clinical trials. The sponsoring company had issued press releases, and information was appearing in the newspapers and on radio and television about a new drug for heart failure. The information about this drug was so positive that one of my patients rushed into my office with a newspaper in his hand and insisted, "Doc, you've got to get this drug for me." He was so caught up in pursuing something newer and bigger and better that he failed to realize that he was already in one of the clinical trials on the drug and had been taking it for the past two years!

But enthusiasm can overtake caution in investigators and administrators as well. One of the new drugs being investigated for the treatment of heart failure was recently shown to be so good in improving patients' exercise tolerance and symptoms that the pharmaceutical company was able to convince the Food and Drug Administration to approve the drug before completion of a study showing whether the drug had an effect on overall mortality in heart failure patients. The drug was released and touted in the media as a major advance in the treatment of heart failure, only to be followed within a month or so by reports from clinical trials revealing increased mortality among patients taking the drug. Probably the only thing worse than building up the hopes of a heart failure patient on the basis of premature claims is to suddenly remove hope.

CURRENT INVESTIGATIONAL DRUG THERAPIES FOR HEART FAILURE

I really cannot give a complete list of investigational treatments for heart failure. First of all, any list would be practically obsolete by the time this book is published, or certainly within a short time thereafter. Furthermore, there are so many areas of development that no list could ever be complete. However, there are several broad areas that have been concentrated on in the recent past. Since we know that the failing heart lacks the power to contract or squeeze, many of the companies developing drugs for heart failure have focused on those that increase the heart's capacity to perform this action. By and large, most of these drugs have produced ill effects. However, there are several new drugs being developed that simulate the heart's squeezing action in a safe and seemingly effective manner. Longer-term studies are under way to determine how long these drugs continue to enhance the contractibility of the heart and to make sure they are safe over a long period of time.

As I discussed earlier, many drug treatments for heart failure work by opening up the arteries and veins, and researchers continuously search for drugs that do so safely, efficiently and, ideally, by means of a once-per-day dosage regimen. Also, researchers are conducting clinical trials to investigate the effects of various combinations of drugs.

ALTERNATIVE DRUGS FOR HEART FAILURE

A recent *New England Journal of Medicine* article estimated that as many as one-third of Americans used some form of alternative health care within the past year, so it would not be surprising to find that many patients with heart failure are looking for alternative measures. I have long been interested in the role of what we call "alternative methods" in all forms of healing. Part of the question, of course, is how you define alternative medicine: For many years, the approach taken by Dr. Dean Ornish—for example, using low-fat diets, exercise, and meditation to help reverse blockages in the coronary arteries—was viewed as an alternative approach. In fact, if you examine carefully some of the alternative methods, they are treatments and approaches that have come down to us from ancient medical systems, and in fact, these methods worked for many cultures for thousands of years. The development of ancient Chinese or Pakistani medicine or Indian Ayurveda came long before our Western ideas about the value of scientific approach of the use of randomized, placebo-controlled clinical trials. Indeed, one of the difficulties we have today is in applying Western scientific methods to these ancient schools of medicine, since the Western approach removes the concept of mind participation in the healing process (or so we think, until we study the importance of placebo effect), whereas the ancient systems actually demand the role of the mind on healing.

At any rate, alternative approaches are becoming more acceptable as mainstream medicine; in fact, insurance companies are beginning to pay for these kinds of treatments. Many good forces are under way to promote a more holistic approach to health and healing, such as the many new journals, for example, *Alternative Therapies in Health and Medicine.* Unfortunately, there is the opportunity for poor practitioners to arise and, as always, they abound. There are now several good books that help the consumer select alternative therapies. Although none is perfect, here are some of the better ones I've read.

- *Alternative Medicine: The Definitive Guide,* by the Burton Goldberg Group (Future Medicine Publishing, 1995).
- *The Alternative Medicine Sourcebook,* by Steven Bratman, M.D. (Lowell House, 1997).
- *Five Steps to Selecting the Best Alternative Medicine,* by Mary Morton and Michael Morton (New York Library, 1996).
- *Natural Medicine for Heart Disease,* by Judith Sachs (Dell Natural Library of Medicine, 1997). This last little book is quite good and balanced in its presentation, and actually gives a great overview of so many approaches and therapies.

As I said, this "alternative and complementary and holistic medicine" concept is booming, and there is so much being published that it is hard to keep up with it all. Usually, most practitioners have their own angle on what works (that is, Rolfing is the answer for all health problems, or juicing cures all, or electromagnetic therapy is the key!). Obviously, a single therapy does not hold all the answers, and, in fact, the key, in my opinion, is good old common sense and prevention. The beauty of this current rage, however, is the ability for patients to realize that their doctors and nurses do not hold all the answers, and, in fact, patients need to do much of the work and take responsibility for their own health and healing. Another positive here is the fact that there may in fact be alternatives to what we have learned in traditional medical school classes. The key is to remain balanced in your approach but keep an open mind.

One of my favorite quotes comes from D. T. Suzuki, who brought Zen Buddhism to the United States at the turn of the century: "In the beginner's mind there are many possibilities, but in the expert's there are few." What this means to me is that we all get so involved in what we have learned that we often are unwilling or unable to accept a new truth or another way of thinking about a problem. The fact is, we all have biases that influence how we make decisions; often, these biases, instead of helping us, put blinders on us or limit our options. Another similar phrase or concept that Dr. Depak Chopra talks about is discussed in the following segment.

"PREMATURE COGNITIVE COMMITMENT"

Again, this concept means that we all form certain biases or prejudices that keep our minds and our thinking locked in rather than allowing us to explore our limitless potentials. The point here is that as patients and healers, it seems to make little sense to apply limits; why should we only choose our treatments and remedies from page one of a multipage menu? We should explore and study the menu, and then choose as wisely as we can.

I recently have been successful in promoting a "cautious look" into complementary and alternative care at a major medical school and hospital system. My hope is that, years from now, all complementary and alternative practices will have become integrative and truly holistic in a greater part of our American health system.

Most alternative approaches to the treatment of heart failure deal with vitamins or minerals, or substances that are purported to have a beneficial effect on the heart—usually with the support of good, hard data to prove the point. Again, I am reluctant to give a catalog of current alternative approaches to treating heart failure, because I am sure there are many I would miss.

Let me talk, however, about one approach in particular that I have advocated and used for more than a decade and that now is getting wider application in our country. The drug, or vitamin really, called ubiquinone, or coenzyme Q_{10}, or CoQ_{10}, has been around for many years and has been touted as improving the energetics of the failing heart. More than any other drug considered an alternative therapy for heart failure, CoQ_{10} has in fact undergone several clinical trials both in the United States and in Europe—with both positive and negative results. One of the problems I see is that most of the clinical trials with CoQ_{10} have not had the firm end points that other trials have, and I think this is certainly something that needs to be addressed. However, when one looks and reads the tremendous bulk of materials available on CoQ_{10}, there really is a strong scientific basis for the use of it in heart failure and many other diseases as well. (See Chapter 19 on the Internet.)

One of the pioneers in studying CoQ_{10} therapy had been Dr. Karl Folkers, whom I have had the privilege to meet and know over the years. Unfortunately, he died in 1997, perhaps just short of the greater acceptance and application of his life's work. I certainly am indebted to him and his career dedication to studying "Q."

As I always tell my patients, another major problem with trying CoQ_{10} therapy, and one I learned about from patients of mine who have wanted to try this therapy, is that this vitamin, which can be bought in health-food stores, is quite expensive and, in fact, can cost as much or more than some of the conventional medications. However, more and more sources for CoQ_{10} appear daily and with a little shopping, a reasonable price can be found.

There are certain heart failure situations in which I almost always recommend CoQ_{10}, such as peripartum cardiomyopathy, alcohol-related heart failure, adriamycin-induced heart failure, and others in which I leave it up to the patient. We should be aware of an interesting finding that the newer drugs we use to lower cholesterol, the so-called "statin" drugs (such as Mevacor, Pravachol, Lipitor, and so on) can actually lower the body's levels of CoQ_{10}. This has led one leading cardiac surgeon to tell me that he expects to see a whole new crop of iatrogenic (disease caused by the doctor or treatment) heart failure to develop. When one thinks about patients at risk for low levels of CoQ_{10}, including the elderly, those with poor nutrition or absorption of nutrients, or chronic diuretic therapy, then supplementation with this vitamin really begins to make sense. Another important aspect is how CoQ_{10} is absorbed into the body, or bioavailability, and some brands (QGel, www.tishcon.com) are absorbed much better. Again, I urge you to read about CoQ_{10}, get a balanced perspective, and discuss it with your doctor. Some good sources for reading include the following:

- *Natural Medicine for Heart Disease,* by Judith Sachs (Dell Natural Library of Medicine, 1997). Again, a good place to start your reading for an overview of many alternative and vitamin therapies.
- *The Miracle Nutrient CoEnzyme Q_{10},* by Emile G. Bliznakov, M.D., and Gerald L. Hunt (Bantam Books, 1987). A good read on the topic, if not well balanced.
- *CoEnzyme Q_{10} and the Heart,* by Stephen T. Sinatra, M.D. (Keats Publishing, 1998).

Again, the Internet is a good place to do your current reading if you enter the net with an open mind and a closed pocketbook.

I am truly hopeful that promising alternative approaches can be investigated in good clinical trials so that their proponents can have the opportunity to establish a sound scientific basis for their claims and to answer the question of whether they are useful approaches for treating patients with heart failure. Hopefully, as the efficacy of alternative treatments is established, they will also become safer and more affordable for patients who need them.

EXPERIMENTAL NONPHARMACOLOGICAL APPROACHES TO TREATING HEART FAILURE

As you have no doubt noticed, most of the attention on treating heart failure, aside from dietary restrictions, has been on using drugs that have one effect or another on the heart. I would like to mention here two nonpharmacological, or nondrug, approaches to treating heart failure that are gaining interest and that you may hear more about in the future.

For years, patients who had heart failure were admonished to not exercise and, in fact, to restrict their lifestyles severely. Although this may reduce the burden on the heart, it also produces a severe deconditioning of the heart, along with the remainder of the muscles in a patient's body. Surprisingly, studies showing the beneficial effects of exercise on patients with heart failure have been conducted only recently. Many heart failure experts now commonly encourage patients to stay as active as possible and, in fact, suggest an aggressive cardiac rehabilitation training program for many. Since many patients with heart failure are elderly and have been severely limited in their exercise abilities for a long time, the period of training or conditioning often takes much longer than would be expected for a sedentary but younger patient. Nevertheless, improvements resulting from exercise training can be seen within a short period of time, and patients may continue to show signs of improvement even after six months or a year. So far, there is no ideal form of exercise, and, surprisingly, even minimal activity has a significant effect on improving a patient's symptoms and ability to exercise.

Since exercise training appears to be quite safe in patients with heart failure and can usually be done without an expensive training program, I think it is one of the modalities we will hear more about and will apply more regularly to patients with advanced heart failure.

Another interesting nondrug way of treating heart failure is through the use of specialized pacemakers called biventricular pacemakers. On the basis of studies first done in Europe, it has been noted that the benefits of pacing the heart muscle to help synchronize contractions of the upper and lower chambers include improving the symptoms of heart failure, exercise tolerance, and perhaps even longer survival time. Several trials have shown that using these biventricular pacemakers patients feel better, can walk farther, and have a better quality of life. Although that alone is terrific, we also feel we need to know if "resynchronization" of the heart using a pacemaker with three leads will actually affect survival. Unfortunately, that answer is not yet in but a couple of trials are getting to the point where we should soon have those answers.

Another question surrounds the treatment of sudden death and one trial is looking at whether a biventricular pacemaker combined with a defibrillator is better than a pacemaker alone or medications alone. Stay tuned for these important results.

As I discuss under Sudden Death in Chapter 17, although we are more clear about who should get a defibrillator for patients with coronary artery disease, we are less clear for patients with normal arteries. This also is an interesting story for which we need answers—I am afraid we will not have a clear picture on this for some time. I think this approach is fascinating, since pacemakers today can be put in quite simply and often do not even require an overnight hospital stay. If there is any evidence that pacemaker therapy works for a significant number of patients with heart failure, I think we will see this becoming a more standard treatment approach, though probably used in conjunction with medication treatments.

As you can see, there are multiple opportunities and options within the experimental approaches for treating heart failure. As each day goes by, better and newer ideas are being developed to help attack the serious problem of heart failure. I think that because of the way research systems operate in the United States, most patients who enter clinical trials are, by and large, allowing themselves the opportunity to try new and potentially groundbreaking treatments while exposing themselves to minimal risk. I think that patients, with the advice and counsel of their physicians, can find the proper match for themselves with an investigational drug or device and thus open up their options for treatment even more.

Even after a patient finds a doctor and center offering investigational therapies, one of the biggest hurdles is often not scaring the patient and family away after they read the legal document called the consent form. Therefore, I found it useful in the original edition of this book, as well as in practice, to let patients and families read a sample consent form and discuss all their questions beforehand.

Finally, there is a terrific little book circulated to physicians and nurses in which a friend of mine, Dr. Robert Kloner, along with Dr. Yochai Birnbaum, compile a listing of many of the current and recently completed clinical trials in cardiovascular disease areas. I do not think this information is well publicized or well summarized anywhere else, but I hope this book will appear electronically somewhere soon.

The following is a sample of a typical consent form provided to my patients for a study we did years ago. The form and some of its content will vary from study to study and between institutions, but it has several of the important elements for your review. The form, however, does not replace a serious discussion with a doctor or nurse involved in the study, a discussion that should address all the issues surrounding the treatment being studied.

CONSENT TO PARTICIPATE IN A RESEARCH STUDY

Metoprolol in Dilated Cardiomyopathy (MDC):
A Randomized Controlled Multicenter Trial

Investigator: Marc A. Silver, M.D.

    Statement of Consent and Purpose of Study: You have a disease of the heart muscle that is called cardiomyopathy. This disease is responsible for symptoms of heart failure, which may include shortness of breath. Cardiomyopathy is a serious disorder that may severely limit a person's endurance or may result in premature death. Currently, there is no medical or surgical cure for this condition. Although conventional treatment is helpful in relieving some of the symptoms, there are certain patients who do not return to a normal or near-normal lifestyle. Some of these patients may benefit from newer forms of treatment.

One of these agents, metoprolol, is in the class of drugs called beta-blockers, which have been used to treat other forms of heart disease. Some patients with cardiomyopathy treated with this drug have had improved exercise tolerance in our experience. Other investigators have confirmed this observation, as well as demonstrated improved survival. Our objectives are to determine how and why patients are improved with metoprolol therapy.

I, _____, voluntarily agree to continue my participation in a research study involving a currently available medication named metoprolol, which is a beta-blocker used to treat high blood pressure, chest pains, and migraine headaches. Its use, however, is experimental in the treatment of cardiomyopathy and heart failure.

Procedures: I agree to take part in a research study that evaluates the action of a drug on my heart. Either metoprolol or placebo (sugar pill) will be selected by lottery for my treatment. The randomization process will be performed by computer from a central location in Sweden. The medication will be started at a very low dose. The dose will be increased eight to ten times over six to eight weeks. After each increase in dose, Dr. Silver or his associates will examine me weekly for the initial six weeks and then at least monthly for twelve months.

Before I am accepted into this study, I will undergo a series of tests to evaluate my heart function to determine if I am eligible to participate in this study. These tests include electrocardiogram, chest X ray, twenty-four-hour Holter (heartbeat recording), echocardiogram (sound wave recording of heart), a MUGA scan, and blood tests (approximately half a tablespoon of blood). Some participants, to make sure they have cardiomyopathy, may have already had a cardiac catheterization, a heart biopsy, or both. I understand that I may be asked to perform a treadmill test prior to the study and again at six and twelve months.

Risks and Discomforts: There are some risks involved in participating in this study. These include adverse effects of metoprolol, all of which are not yet known. The known side effects include, in some patients, a worsening of their shortness of breath or an accumulation of fluid. This usually responds to decreasing the dose of metoprolol or increasing the dose of water pills. More often, some patients may feel tired or listless and may experience mild gastrointestinal problems, slowing of the heart rate, lowered blood pressure, or wheezing. I realize that metoprolol is still an investigational drug for my condition and that unexpected side effects could occur.

Benefits: It is possible that my continuing participation in this investigation may be beneficial and that if I continue to take metoprolol, my symptoms of heart failure may improve, as has been seen with other patients.

Alternative Procedures: Alternative medical therapy approved for the treatment of my heart failure, and which may be chosen if I decide not to participate in this study, consists of noninvestigational drugs, such as captopril.

Confidentiality of Data: I hereby agree to allow my name and medical records to be made available to Dr. Silver and to the Food and Drug Administration for the purpose of evaluating the results of his study. I consent to the publication of any data that may result from this study provided my name and any identifying information is not included in such publication. Therefore, information that may be identified with me will be released only with my written permission or as required by law.

Compensation for Injury: I understand that in the event of physical injury resulting from the research procedures the hospital will provide me with free emergency care, if such care is necessary. I also understand that if I wish, the hospital will provide nonemergency medical care but that neither Dr. Silver nor the hospital assumes any responsibility to pay for such care or to provide me with financial compensation.

Costs: I understand that my participation in this research is not expected to result in any additional costs to me beyond what could be normally expected for treatment of my condition.

Absence of Guarantee: Dr. Silver has not made or represented any guarantee to me as to the results that I may expect from participation in this study.

Right to Withdraw: I have been advised that Dr. Marc A. Silver will answer any questions I may have regarding this research study, research-related injury, and research subject rights; that I am free to withdraw my consent and discontinue participation at any time without penalty; and that standard medical treatment for my condition will remain available to me. I have also been advised that Dr. Silver may terminate my participation in the study if in his judgment this action would be in my best interest.

If I choose to withdraw from this study, I agree to consult with Dr. Silver regarding the consequences of my decision and to let him conduct an orderly termination procedure for ending my participation in this study.

Dr. Silver can be reached by telephone at the following numbers:

_____

_____

Any significant new findings that develop during the course of this research that may be related to me will be provided to me.

I have been given a copy of this consent form, I have read and understood it, and I have had my questions answered.

_____

Patient's signature

_____

Witness's Name

_____

Witness's Signature

_____

Date

11

Food and Heart Failure

When patients who have read the first edition of this book talk with me or write to me, the one chapter they have commented on the most is the chapter on food and the sodium content. It is interesting, since I actually almost did not include this chapter in the first edition. Now, I would not even think about not including it. I have left it basically untouched in this edition. Many readers were able to peruse the sodium contents and realize how many foods fooled them into thinking they were healthy or okay to eat. I have made little in the way of additions to this chapter. However, on a recent trip to McDonald's with my children (okay, yes, I went but didn't swallow), I asked for an updated *McDonald's Nutrition Facts*. Very interesting reading. Pick one up on your next visit to McDonald's, Burger King, Arby's, and so on.

It is really from the knowledge of the many concerned dietitians whom I have worked with over the years and of my superb nursing clinicians—all of whom seem to spend half their waking hours checking out the food labels in grocery stores and the menus of restaurants—that I have compiled most of this information. Since one of my primary goals is to get heart failure patients back to a more active, productive, and normal lifestyle, and since that lifestyle includes dining out for many people, I am including in this chapter information on eating in restaurants, working lunches, and sharing meals with family and friends that will not cause regrets later. This information is certainly not meant to be totally inclusive, but it includes some of the common tips we pass on to our patients, advice I think all Americans would do well to heed. (There are excellent resources that address the issue of food and the heart, and many are mentioned in Appendix II.)

WHERE'S THE SALT?

There is a lot of confusion as to what exactly sodium or salt is. Sodium is a naturally occurring mineral and, as such, is found in a variety of the foods we eat as well as in many other sources, including medications, drinks, and even softened water. Salt is sodium combined with chloride, another mineral. By and large, the table salt we eat is about 40 percent sodium and 60 percent chloride. Most people get most of their sodium from salt. Sodium is absolutely essential for regulating many of the activities of the body and for keeping the fluid balance normal. We all need a certain amount of salt in our diet each day. It is estimated that the average person needs less than 500 milligrams of sodium per day, or approximately one-fourth of a teaspoon of salt. Unfortunately, most Americans end up consuming as much as 5,000 or 6,000 milligrams of salt on a daily basis. Some experts recommend that the average American ingest no more than 3,000 milligrams of sodium per day, and, in fact, I tell most of my patients with heart failure that they should have no more than 2,000 milligrams a day (or even less for certain people).

I will discuss some of the foods that contain salt or sodium and some of the hidden sources of sodium, but for many people there really is no mystery as to why they consume 3,000 to 5,000 milligrams of sodium on a daily basis. In fact, the answer is in their hands. These people are the heavy salt users, and we've all seen them; they are the ones who salt their food even before they taste it. This is a very bad habit, one that is commonly learned growing up, and it can cause all kinds of medical problems, including high blood pressure. One way people who have heart failure and who need to restrict their salt or sodium intake each day can make a major impact on their health is simply to limit use of the saltshaker. By adding no salt with a saltshaker, people can usually reduce their sodium content by as much as one-third or more of their daily intake. People frequently ask me if they can use a salt substitute instead of the saltshaker. If you read the labels of most salt substitutes, you will find that they contain other chlorides, such as potassium chloride, which are also salts. A high intake of potassium can send the body's potassium balance out of whack, particularly if a person is taking drugs, such as any one of the ACEIs, which have a tendency to make the body retain potassium. For those who are taking diuretics that tend to make the body hold on to potassium, the use of such a salt substitute can really cause a serious, even life-threatening, problem. I therefore tell most of my patients to get in the habit of living without a saltshaker; usually, over a period of one or two months, they are able to adjust to a diet with a lower sodium content.

SALT BY ANY OTHER NAME . . .

One of the things people with heart failure have to learn to do is to look at the labels of all the food they eat or buy in the store to better determine the sodium content. Today, foods are increasingly labeled with nutritional information, including the exact milligram content of sodium in the food either per container or per serving, but this does not apply to every food. Clearly, when the label says salt, most people are aware that this means this food has a certain amount of sodium in it. But what if the label says sodium alginate or sodium sulfite, or sodium caseinate or disodium phosphate, or sodium benzoate or sodium hydroxide? These are all forms of sodium! Many of them are preservatives that are used in the foods, but they still count toward your daily sodium intake. Everyone is aware of monosodium glutamate, or MSG, which is commonly used as a seasoning in Chinese foods, but many people are not aware that other forms of sodium, such as sodium citrate (which is used as an antioxidant in baking), can cause similar problems. Careful attention to food labels, as well as more pressure from Americans to have foods labeled more completely and properly, will make the whole process of monitoring sodium intake simpler in the future.

IT'S A JUNGLE OUT THERE

Manufacturers of processed foods have been quick to pick up on this interest of the American public in restricting sodium or salt in their diet. But it seems that rather than make an earnest effort to help Americans restrict the salt in their diet, manufacturers have come up with various terms that seem to confuse people more than anything else. The word *light* or *lite* is being used almost everywhere, and poor, unsuspecting Americans are gobbling up these foods and imaging that they are getting lighter in weight and healthier with every bite. By and large, these "light" foods contain a smaller percentage of calories than an equivalent portion of a comparable product, but they make no other specific claims, particularly with regard to sodium content. In fact, some of the "light" products contain the highest sodium content I've seen around!

Another term that is being used is *low sodium,* and this generally refers to products that contain less than 140 milligrams of sodium per serving, or per 100 grams of food. Although these are generally better than equivalent products that are not low in sodium, consumers must recognize that they can still get into a lot of trouble eating just a few servings of these low-sodium foods. The designation salt-free means that the food product contains less than 5 milligrams of sodium per serving. This truly is a restricted sodium food and probably is better than either the low-sodium or full-sodium products.

Since Americans get over 80 percent of the sodium they ingest each day from processed foods, it is almost better to stay away from processed foods altogether. For example, many of my patients make their own soups at home with no added salt, using only vegetables and chicken or meat. An eight-ounce bowl of home-made soup with no salt added either in the cooking process or at the table has no more than about 25–30 milligrams of sodium. But just half a can of a certain brand of processed chicken noodle soup has well over 1,000 milligrams of sodium. As a general rule, fresh fruits and vegetables and foods that are prepared in the home are far better for you than most processed foods or most restaurant foods.

Among common foods that many Americans seem to have trouble with are bread products. I learned an important lesson two years ago when my wife and I bought a home bread machine for a Christmas present. We went to the bookstore and bought a wonderful book of recipes on making breads in our new machine. We were shocked, however, when we saw how much salt was added to most regular bread recipes. We gradually cut back further and further, until we added no salt at all to the recipes, and—lo and behold—they tasted just as good and came out just as well. I think learning to live without salt in the diet is like most other conditions in life: One can grow accustomed to it in a relatively short period of time. In our home, we do not have a saltshaker on the table—in fact, I haven't even seen it in well over two years! Our children do not use salt, and although they do like some salty snacks, they limit their consumption of them to rare occasions.

Another step to take is to learn which foods are high in sodium and which ones are low. For example, foods that are generally high in sodium—and by that, I mean containing over 150 milligrams per serving—are, almost without exception, lunch meats (such as bologna or salami), hot dogs, bacon, cheese, canned soups, crackers, and pretzels. A good rule of thumb is to buy frozen instead of canned vegetables, because salt is usually used as a preservative in the canning process. On the other hand, foods that have a lower sodium content, usually no more than 50 milligrams per serving, are fresh vegetables, fresh fruit, and pasta that has been cooked with little or no sodium in the water. And, yes, you can even eat popcorn that has not been salted.

BETTER SALT SUBSTITUTES

Whether it is truly a matter of taste or psychological, getting rid of all the salty flavor is too much for some people to bear. Fortunately, there are some excellent herbs and spices that are good alternatives for flavoring food, including some commercially prepared brands, such as Mrs. Dash and Papa Dash. However, I commonly tell people to use generous amounts of lemon juice or vinegar, particularly on vegetables and salads. Meats and vegetables can be cooked with mushrooms, mint leaves, green peppers, or even generous amounts of onions and garlic. Even cooking with fruit, for example, apricots and peaches, is an option. One of my patients became almost addicted to fresh horseradish when he found that it was the only thing that would allow him to beat the salt habit.

Go to your spice shelf and look at all those little bottles of spices you may have bought years ago and have never known what to do with. These spices can now become good substitutes for salt. Many of them—such as allspice, bay leaves, caraway seeds, garlic powder, marjoram, dry mustard, thyme, ginger, paprika, rosemary, sage, tarragon, basil, dill, and poppy seeds—can be used either at the table or during cooking to enhance the flavor of your food and get you out of the salt habit. Talk to your local nutritionist or your hospital dietitian for other suggestions on what to substitute for the high salt-containing foods in your diet.

THE BIG HITTERS

Not too long ago, a patient with whom my staff and I had spent a fair amount of time in the office going over salt and fluid restriction, as we normally do, decided that he wanted to tell me exactly what he had eaten one day on the previous weekend. Actually, I think he just wanted to see how much I could cringe. For lunch he went to a fast-food restaurant and ate a quarter-pound hamburger with cheese plus a half-dozen dill pickles (the friends he ate with disliked the dill pickles that came on their sandwiches and gave them to my patient). He assured me that the pickles couldn't have been a problem because the fast-food chain was getting so cheap that they were slicing the pickles very thin. Unfortunately, the burger with cheese contained well over 1,100 milligrams of sodium, and when I told my patient that the dill pickles probably had the same amount of sodium as the entire hamburger, he thought I was simply picking on him. He thought I would be pleased to hear that for dinner he had chicken. Unfortunately, this was not a grilled or broiled breast of chicken but the Colonel's original-recipe fried chicken. I estimated that his serving probably added another 2,000 milligrams of sodium to his total for the day.

There are other foods that are also "big hitters" in the sodium league that you might not be aware of. One cup of potato salad can have as much as 1,300 milligrams of sodium, a chef's salad with ham and cheese on top can have 1,100 or 1,200, and spaghetti with meat sauce can have 1,000. Just to give you an idea of the range in the sodium content of foods, here are two tables, one (Table 11.1) listing some foods that have either a low or medium sodium content and the other (Table 11.2) listing those with a high sodium content.

TABLE 11.1 Foods with a Low to Medium Sodium Content

Food	Milligrams of sodium
Apple	2
Applesauce (1 cup)	6
Bread (one slice/white)	114
Butter (1 tbsp, salted)	116
Club soda (8 oz)	39
Fresh tuna (3 oz)	50
Margarine (1 tbsp)	140
Tomato	14
Water (8 oz tap)	12
White wine (4 oz)	19

Source: U.S. Department of Agriculture.

Table 11.3 lists a number of obvious and perhaps not so obvious foods with a high sodium content. It would be wise to try to avoid these "big hitters."

DINING OUT

Without a doubt, my patients who eat more than one or two meals in a restaurant each week have the most difficult time controlling their consumption of sodium. People eat meals out nowadays for a variety of reasons. Some are busy and don't have time to prepare foods in their homes. I've been told that up to 60 percent of Americans eat lunch in a fast-food restaurant, a dramatic shift even in the past decade. One of my patients is quite poor and lives in a YMCA hotel; he has no cooking facilities there and must eat all of his meals out, which means that it has been extremely hard for him to control the salt in his diet. Because of either their inability or an unwillingness to cook, the elderly tend to eat a lot of meals in restaurants (and very commonly in fast-food restaurants because of the cost).

Whatever their reasons for frequently dining out, all patients with heart failure have to be aware that restaurants, particularly fast-food restaurants, are danger signs along the road to feeling better. The following are some tips you would be wise to follow when you eat out at a restaurant:

1. Before you go to the restaurant, try to find out if they serve a wide variety of foods rather than a specific form of food. For example, going to a restaurant that serves only deep-fried items is going to be a disaster. You might want to call ahead and see if they have the American Heart Association's Heart Healthy Diets on their menu. A quick call to the restaurant, even anonymously, can save you embarrassment once you're there and discomfort after you've eaten your meal there.

2. Once you get to the restaurant, take your time and look carefully at the menu. Be sure to ask the waiter or waitress how the food is prepared if you are in doubt. Ask the waitperson for low-sodium suggestions; trust me, they have been asked before! See if foods can be prepared without salt, and choose foods with the lowest sodium content.

3. As an appetizer, get either a fruit-containing item, fruit juice, or a vegetable, rather than a pasta or baked item.

4. For your entree, order something that can be roasted, broiled, or grilled without adding extra salt. Fish or fresh meats are good choices. Pasta—if you can get it without the sauce, say with a little garlic and oil—is probably better for you than something like a breaded veal cutlet.

5. Avoid sauces and gravies at all costs. They are usually high in sodium and will only get you into trouble. Also avoid breaded items, which are also high in salt or sodium content. When you order a salad, try to use a low-sodium salad dressing, if one is available, or—better yet—use vinegar and oil on your salad. And try to use the separate vinegar and oil containers rather than the combinations, which may be commercially prepared and may have a high sodium content.

What should you do if all else fails and you're in a situation where there's virtually nothing on the menu that you can eat that does not have some sodium in it? I recommend that you simply cut down on your portion size and realize that for the next day or so, your sodium restriction is going to have to be even more strict. Despite all that, I must say that eating out today is easier for the heart failure patient than it was before because of the acceptance of patrons' dietary restrictions and the flexibility of most restaurants. I think it helps most, however, to be thoroughly familiar with foods that are high in sodium, so that you can avoid them and make more intelligent selections from a menu.

TABLE 11.2 Foods with High Sodium Content

Food	Milligrams of sodium
Antacid in water	564
Apple pie (⅛ cup)	108
Canned tuna (3 oz)	384
Corn flakes (1 cup)	256
Cottage cheese (4 oz)	457
Dill pickle	928
English muffin	293
Salt (1 tsp)	1,938
Soy sauce (1 tbsp)	1,029
Tomato soup (1 cup)	932

Source: U.S. Department of Agriculture.

TABLE 11.3 Where the Sodium Is: The Big Hitters

Food	Milligrams in sodium
10¾ oz serving Campbell's Chunky Chicken Noodle Soup	1,140
1 McDonald's quarter pounder with cheese	1,110
4 oz Kellogg's All-Bran, dry	1,040
1 cup Jell-O Instant Chocolate Pudding	1,030
1 (6½ oz) can Chicken of the Sea Chunk Light Tuna in Spring Water, drained	994
1 Stouffer's French Bread Deluxe Pizza	950
1 tbsp Kikkoman Soy Sauce	938
1 medium dill pickle	928
1 Hardee's chef's salad, without dressing	910
2 oz Kraft Velveeta	860
1 cube Wyler Chicken Flavor Bouillon	850
½ cup Chef Boyardee Spaghetti Sauce with Mushrooms	845
3 Bisquick Original Mix pancakes	700
½ cup cooked Uncle Ben's Brown or Wild Rice	500
4 oz Light n' Lively Free Cottage Cheese	390
1 (4.3 oz) Hostess Apple Pie	370
1 tbsp Dijon mustard	360
3 cups Orville Redenbacher Natural Flavor Popcorn (for microwave)	330

Presented in Table 11.4 are some of the foods typically eaten for breakfast, lunch, and dinner in restaurants (or, for that matter, at home), along with their sodium content. Table 11.5 lists selections from the major sections of a restaurant menu that are recommended and those you are advised to avoid.

Since many of our patients do eat in fast-food restaurants, in Table 11.6, I "name names" and show you exactly what the sodium content is for most of these foods. As you can see, there are very few low-sodium foods you can get in a fast-food restaurant.

Food plays an important role in our lives; we eat not only for sustenance but also to fulfill social and business rites. Many patients develop heart disease due, in part, to their dietary habits. In general, something that is restricted takes on more attention and importance, but I believe that most patients can and do readily adapt to a low-sodium diet. For some patients, following charts and recipes is the only way to maintain the diet; others grasp the general notion and can stay well within their limits on a daily basis. It is critical, however, for patients and families to accept the necessity of dietary restrictions based on an understanding of the disease. Finally, patients and their families must make sure that the diet does not control them or adversely affect their lives and, instead, should take the perspective that diet is yet another aspect of life that they can control, enjoy, and from which they can benefit.

TABLE 11.4 Sodium Content of Common Foods

Food item	Milligrams of sodium
Breakfast	
Bacon, pork (2 strips)	202
Bagel with 1 oz cream cheese	283
Bran muffin	168
Coffee, brewed (1 cup)	8
Coffee cake (1 piece)	310
Cornflakes (1 cup) with low-fat milk	361
Corn muffin	192
Danish pastry, plain	249
Doughnut, plain	139
English muffin	358
French toast (2 slices)	514
Fried egg, large (1)	162
Fruit yogurt, low-fat (1 cup)	133
Grapefruit, half	0
Hash browns (1 cup)	54
Link sausages, pork (2)	336
Oatmeal, cooked (1 cup)	1
Orange juice, frozen (1 cup)	2
Pancakes (2)	320
Tea, brewed (1 cup)	8
Toast, wheat (1 slice)	153
Tomato juice, canned (1 cup)	882
Two-egg omelet, ham and cheese	598
Lunch	
Cheeseburger, fast food	750
Cheese pizza (1 slice)	261
Chef's salad, ham and cheese (1 cup)	1,134
Chicken noodle soup (1 cup)	1,107
Chicken noodle soup, low-sodium (1 cup)	36
Cola (12 oz)	12
Coleslaw (1/2 cup)	16
Corn chips (1 oz)	164
Cottage cheese, low-fat (1 cup)	918
Diet cola (12 oz)	24
Dill pickle (1 medium)	928
French fries (20), unsalted	30
Fruit salad (1 cup)	9
Green salad, tossed (1 cup)	53
Ham and cheese sandwich	792
Hamburger, fast food	500
Hot dog on bun	671
Potato chips (14 chips)	164
Potato salad (1 cup)	1,323
Roast beef sandwich	792

(continued)

Table 11.4 (*Continued*)

Food item	Milligrams of sodium
Lunch (cont.)	
Tomato, whole (1)	10
Tuna salad (1 cup)	434
Vegetable beef soup (1 cup)	957
Vegetable soup, low-sodium (1 cup)	38
Dinner	
Beef burrito, fast food	746
Beef or pork chop suey, homemade (1 cup)	1,052
Beer (12 oz)	24
Broccoli, raw/boiled (1 cup)	16
Broiled codfish (1 fillet)	141
Broiled pork chop	49
Broiled sirloin steak (4 oz)	74
Chicken chow mein, homemade (1 cup)	717
Chili con carne (1 cup)	135
Dinner roll	144
Fettuccine Alfredo, frozen (1 portion)	1,195
Fish sticks (4 oz)	651
Fried chicken breast	385
Green beans, french, frozen (1 cup)	17
Light beer (12 oz)	12
Macaroni and cheese, homemade (1 cup)	1,086
Peas and carrots, frozen/boiled (1 cup)	110
Potato, peeled and boiled	7
Red wine (4 oz)	76
Rice, cooked (1 cup)	4
Roast chicken breast	138
Roast turkey breast, without skin (1 cup)	89
Spaghetti with tomato-meat sauce (1 cup)	1,009
White wine (4 oz)	72
Desserts	
Angel food cake (1 slice)	142
Apple pie (1 slice)	207
Banana	1
Brownie with nuts (1)	50
Cheesecake (1 slice)	189
Chocolate chip cookies (2)	76
Chocolate pudding (1 cup)	335
Devil's food cake with chocolate icing (1 slice)	180
Fresh pineapple (1 cup)	1
Fresh strawberries (1 cup)	2
Hot fudge sundae (2 scoops)	190
Lemon meringue pie (1 slice)	223
Oatmeal-raisin cookies (2)	74
Orange sherbet (½ cup)	44
Pound cake (1 slice)	58

(*continued*)

TABLE 11.4 (*Continued*)

Food item	Milligrams of sodium
Desserts (cont.)	
Rice pudding with raisins (1 cup)	188
Vanilla ice cream (½ cup)	58
Yellow cake with white icing (1 slice)	191
Condiments	
Barbecue sauce (¼ cup)	508
Brown gravy (¼ cup)	31
Butter, regular (1 pat)	41
Butter, unsalted (1 pat)	< 1
Catsup (1 tbsp)	156
Cream cheese (1 tbsp)	85
Hollandaise sauce (¼ cup)	284
Italian dressing (1 tbsp)	116
Italian dressing, low-calorie (1 tbsp)	118
Margarine (1 pat)	47
Mayonnaise (1 tbsp)	104
Mushroom gravy (¼ cup)	340
Mustard, prepared (1 tbsp)	195
Pancake syrup (2 tbsp)	70
Parmesan cheese (1 tbsp)	116
Soy sauce (1 tbsp)	1,029
Thousand Island dressing (1 tbsp)	109
Thousand Island dressing, low-calorie (1 tbsp)	153
White sauce (¼ cup)	199
Worcestershire sauce (1 tbsp)	147

TABLE 11.5 Dining Out: What to Order and What to Avoid

Menu section	Recommended	Not recommended (too high in fat and/or sodium)
Appetizers	Fruit juice	Soups, especially cream style
	Fresh or canned fruit	Fried vegetables or potato skins
	Gelatin	Vegetable juices
	Relish plates (with raw vegetables)	Relish plates (with preserved or pickled items)
Salads	Fresh vegetable salad served with lemon, vinegar, or low-calorie dressing	Coleslaw
	Sliced tomatoes	Macaroni or potato salad
	Fruit salad	Salad with excessive amounts of salad dressing
	Gelatin salad	Cottage cheese

(*continued*)

TABLE 11.5 (*Continued*)

Menu section	Recommended	Not recommended (too high in fat and/or sodium)
Entrees	Any lean meat, fish, or poultry that has been roasted, baked, boiled, or poached	Stews and casserole-type dishes
		Fatty, fried, or breaded meats
		Eggs
Vegetables	Stewed, steamed, or boiled	Those in a sauce or au gratin
		Seasoned with butter or cooked in egg yolk batter
		Fried vegetables
Potatoes and substitutes	Mashed, baked, boiled, or steamed potatoes	Fried potatoes
	Boiled or steamed rice	Creamed or au gratin potatoes
	Boiled noodles	Fried rice
		Noodles in a cream sauce
Breads	Hard or soft rolls	Crescents, butter rolls, popovers, and croissants
	Plain bread or toast	Sweet rolls, cakes, or coffee cake
	Unsalted crackers	Salted crackers or breads
	Breadsticks or melba toast	
	Matzos and plain toast	
Condiments	Low-calorie salad dressing	Excess gravy
	Oil and vinegar (use oil sparingly)	Fried or creamed items
		Butter or cream
		Sour cream
		Cream cheese
		Bacon
		Mayonnaise-type salad dressing
		Cheese sauces
Desserts	Fresh fruit	Pastries, cakes, and cream pies
	Angel food cake	Chocolate
	Sherbet or Italian ice	Ice cream
	Fruit sorbet or frozen nonfat or lowfat yogurt	
	Ice milk	
	Gelatin	
Beverages	Fruit juices	Milk shakes
	Skim milk	Chocolate milk
	Soft drinks	Whole milk
	Tea or coffee, preferably decaffeinated	Cocoa
		Alcohol (unless allowed by physician)

TABLE 11.6 Sodium Content of Fast Food

Menu item	Portion	Milligrams of sodium
Kentucky Fried Chicken		
Original Recipe		
Wing	1	387
Center breast	1	532
Drumstick	1	269
Thigh	1	517
Extra-Crispy Recipe		
Wing	1	437
Center breast	1	842
Drumstick	1	346
Thigh	1	766
Buttermilk biscuits	1	521
Mashed potatoes with gravy	1	297
Coleslaw	1	171
McDonald's		
Egg McMuffin	1	740
Hot cakes with butter and syrup	1	640
Scrambled eggs	1	290
Pork sausage	1	350
Hash brown potatoes	1	330
Biscuit with sausage and egg	1	1,250
Hamburger	1	500
Cheeseburger	1	750
Quarter Pounder	1	718
Big Mac	1	950
Filet-O-Fish	1	1,030
McDLT	1	990
Chicken McNuggets	6 pieces	520
Chef salad	1	490
Chunky chicken salad	1	230
French fries	1 small	110
Apple pie	1	240
Vanilla shake	1	170
Chocolate shake	1	240
Strawberry shake	1	170
McDonaldland cookies	1	300
Chocolate chip cookies	1	280
Pizza Hut		
(All portions are based on two slices of medium pizza.)		
Pan Pizza		
Cheese		940
Pepperoni		1,127
Supreme		1,363
Super Supreme		1,447

(continued)

TABLE 11.6 (*Continued*)

Menu item	Portion	Milligrams of sodium
Pizza Hut (*cont.*)		
Thin 'n Crispy Pizza		
Cheese		867
Pepperoni		867
Supreme		1,328
Super Supreme		1,336
Personal Pan Pizza		
Pepperoni	1 whole	1,335
Supreme	1 whole	1,313
Subway		
Subway Club	1	839
Turkey Sub	1	839
Tuna Sub	1	905
Steak Sub	1	883
Meatball Sub	1	876
Ham Sub	1	839
Roast Beef Sub	1	839
Seafood and Crab Sub	1	1,306
Subway chef salad without dressing	1	479
Taco Bell		
Taco	1	276
Taco Light	1	594
Soft Taco	1	516
Soft Taco Supreme	1	516
Tostada	1	596
Taco salad with salsa	1	1,286
Taco salad without shell	1	1,056
Steak fajitas	1	485
Chicken fajitas	1	619
Wendy's		
Omelet #3: Ham, cheese, onion, green pepper	1	485
Omelet #4: Mushroom, onion, green pepper	1	200
Breakfast sandwich	1	770
French toast	2 slices	850
¼ lb single hamburger on white bun	1	360
¼ lb bacon cheeseburger on white bun	1	780
Frosty (medium)	12 oz	220
Plain baked potato	1	60
Baked potato with chili and cheese	1	610
White Castle		
Hamburger	1	266
Cheeseburger	1	361
Fish sandwich without tartar sauce	1	201
Chicken sandwich	1	497
Sausage and egg sandwich	1	698
Sausage sandwich	1	488

(*continued*)

TABLE 11.6 (*Continued*)

Menu item	Portion	Milligrams of sodium
Arby's		
Roast beef	1	588
Beef and cheddar	1	955
Ham and cheese	1	1,350
Chicken breast sandwich	1	1,082
Turkey deluxe	1	1,047
Potato cakes	1	397
Burger King		
Breakfast Croissan'wich Cheese	1	607
Breakfast Croissan'wich Bacon	1	719
Breakfast Croissan'wich Sausage	1	985
Breakfast Croissan'wich Ham	1	962
Scrambled egg platter		
Egg, croissant, hash browns	1	893
Egg, with sausage	1	1,271
Egg, with bacon	1	1,043
French toast sticks	1	537
Great Danish	1	288
Bagel sandwich		
Egg and cheese	1	759
Egg and bacon	1	872
Egg and sausage	1	1,137
Egg and ham	1	1,114
Milk, 2%	8 oz	122
Milk, whole	8 oz	119
Whopper	1	865
Whopper with Cheese	1	1,177
Bacon Double Cheeseburger	1	748
Mushroom Swiss Double Burger	1	795
Hamburger	1	505
Cheeseburger	1	661
Cheeseburger Deluxe	1	652
Hamburger Deluxe	1	496
Chicken Broiler Sandwich	1	746
Chicken Tenders	1	54
Chef salad	1	568
Chicken Chunky Salad	1	443
Thousand Island dressing	2 oz	403
French dressing	2 oz	400
Ranch dressing	2 oz	316
Olive oil and vinegar	2 oz	214
Reduced-calorie Italian dressing	2 oz	762

12

Other Forms of
Treatment for Heart Failure

In previous chapters, I discussed conventional as well as experimental treatments for heart failure and addressed the topic of heart transplantation. These are the primary medical and surgical approaches to treating patients with heart failure. In this chapter, I want to talk about several additional treatments: a drug treatment that is given in an intermittent form either in the patient's home or in an outpatient setting, such as a heart failure center or hospital. Later in the chapter, I discuss some important adjunctive treatments for heart failure: surgical treatments and other investigational treatments as well as a few basics including supplemental oxygen and elastic support stockings.

INTERMITTENT INFUSIONS

Many years ago, one of my patients was having difficulty being weaned off an intravenous medicine that he was getting to strengthen his heart while he waited for a heart transplant. We convinced one of the home care agencies that it was perfectly safe for this man to get the treatments in his home, since he had not had any problems in the hospital and this was the only thing preventing him from spending time at home with his family. It worked, and so began my interest in using infusions of heart-strengthening medicines in alternative settings other than in the hospital.

One of the treatments your doctor may use when your heart muscle gets particularly weak is intravenous administration of a drug to help the heart pump stronger. Several such drugs are on the market, including dobutamine, amrinone, and milrinone. A newer drug called Natrecor (neseritide) has just become available and in many cases is the superior drug to use as an intravenous drug and so I will discuss it more fully at the end of this section. One or more of these might well be the drug your doctor would turn to should you be admitted to the hospital with serious heart failure and retaining large amounts of fluid. Helping the heart to pump stronger, these drugs work with diuretics to help clear your body of the excess fluid you are retaining; they may well make you feel better rapidly, and they certainly help to compensate your heart failure. Although some patients need to get these drugs on a continuous basis to be able to go home from the hospital, it is more common today for doctors to use these drugs in an intermittent fashion for patients who are frequently admitted to the hospital to clear the fluid from their body. A doctor may decide to use intermittent infusion with a patient who is on a downward course, for example, one who has had one or two heart failure admissions over the past couple of years, who is now beginning to retain more fluid despite increasing doses of the diuretics, and who has had perhaps increasing hospital admissions over a period of months. One of the doctor's goals is certainly to improve how the patient feels; another is to limit the number of hospitalizations. Thus, the doctor may choose to give this patient intermittent infusions of drugs to help control the heart failure—in a sense, to prevent marked worsening of the heart failure—and to therefore prevent recurrent hospitalizations.

Let me say at the outset that despite increasingly widespread use of these intermittent infusions, there has been no evidence that they prolong the lives of patients who have serious heart failure. A patient who is at the point of requiring frequent infusions has very advanced heart failure; obviously, the long-term prognosis may not be good. On the other hand, I think doctors who have had broad experience using infusions feel that this procedure does certainly limit the number of recurrent hospitalizations and that it can support a patient during a difficult period (when there is more heart failure) and allow the physician to try other therapies afterward that may even allow the patient to come off the infusions completely.

There are many issues regarding the use and abuse of intravenous infusions of inotropic (that is, affecting muscle contractility) drugs, issues that are still being sorted out in the professional literature. However, I think that there are some common issues of which patients should be aware.

There are two common drug types that are used for these kinds of infusions. But also see the update on Natrecor at the end of this section. It will certainly be up to your doctor to decide which one is best for you, but I think one of the important aspects of these infusion treatments is that the choice of drug be made in a more or less scientific fashion. Under the best circumstances, the drug chosen will be one that has definitely been shown to improve a particular individual's heart function. There is a lot of variability in patients' responses to these drugs; that is, a drug may work perfectly well for one patient but not at all for another. Commonly, we test the drugs when a patient is hospitalized and has a Swan-Ganz catheter in place, which can tell us about how the heart and lung pressures respond to a dose of a drug. We also know, however, that a patient's acute response in the hospital may not predict his or her more chronic response after leaving the hospital. In fact, a patient who responds well to Drug X in the hospital may later cease to respond to that drug. Nonetheless, testing the drug while the patient is hospitalized with a Swan-Ganz catheter in place is very useful in determining which drug he or she should get as an outpatient.

Another valid way to select the right drug to use is to observe what we call the "clinical response," that is, the patient's response to an intervention, which in this case is how well the patient gets rid of fluid while he or she is on the drug. However, when patients are hospitalized, they receive several therapies at one time, including diuretics, bed rest, and salt and fluid restriction, recommendations to which they may not have strictly adhered at home. These therapies may falsely lead the physician to believe that it is the particular intravenous drug that is working wonders for the patient when, in fact, the patient's improvement may be due to the enforced adherence to these basic components of conventional care. Nevertheless, most physicians can determine when a drug has accelerated or improved the patient's course and can use that clinical information to decide which drug the patient should receive for further infusions.

Unfortunately, not all physicians are familiar with how to administer and assess the effects of these kinds of drugs, and some end up using only what they are most familiar with or learned about during their training. I believe that this is unfair to the patient; as I said earlier, there should be some scientific basis for choosing a particular drug. You should also know that this is a rather controversial area, and that there are some physicians who feel that there is no clear role for these intravenous drugs.

HOW OFTEN TO GET THE TREATMENTS AND FOR HOW LONG

Another rather unclear area regarding infusions is how long the outpatient's intermittent infusions should be. Normally, when patients are in the hospital, they get these intravenous inotropic drugs continuously for one or more days, but at some point, a decision has to be made about how often individuals should get them as outpatients and with what frequency. Most patients end up getting the infusions once per week, or at most, two or three times per week. This is a somewhat arbitrary decision, but it is one that should be based on the particular patient's ability to be weaned off the drug prior to discharge from the hospital, as well as on frequent clinical assessment by the physician. If a patient is able to come off a drug completely and leave the hospital, but the physician is concerned that he or she may need the drug again to prevent a recurrence of the heart failure, then it will be necessary to check the patient quite closely, even within a day or two after discharge from the hospital. If there are early signs of reaccumulation of fluid (weight gain or increased shortness of breath), the patient may be a candidate for infusion at least once or twice during the subsequent week to prevent rehospitalization. Some patients need infusions almost constantly, and in those situations, everything should be done to try to improve the patient's overall status. Other patients end up getting infusions approximately once a week and then after a period of stability are weaned down to once every other week, with some patients getting by with infusions once every three or four weeks. In my general experience, once patients can be weaned down to once every other week, they usually tell you that they don't feel much different after the infusions; at that point, the procedure can be discontinued, either on a permanent or a temporary basis.

Another decision to make involves the duration of an individual infusion procedure. I've seen infusions given for anywhere from three to about seventy-four hours, with some physicians in the latter case admitting their patients on a Friday afternoon and keeping them until late in the day on Sunday for what they call an "inotrope holiday." I think this extended infusion should be reserved for the most refractory of patients. It certainly sounds like anything but a holiday to me! I generally give my patients about six hours of treatment when they need it, since that tends to work out well from a scheduling perspective and also, I think, allows an ample infusion of the medication. Shorter periods do not give ample time for the drug to give its full benefit. However, I admit that decisions about infusions are purely judgment calls; there's little technical information to say that one protocol or duration is better than another.

WHERE INFUSIONS ARE GIVEN

As I mentioned earlier, infusions can be given with patients being either temporary inpatients in the hospital or outpatients at home or in a variety of settings. Many hospitals have patients come in for a stay of four, six, or eight hours in their emergency department or on one of the telemetry (monitoring) floors. I have those sorts of telemetry outpatient arrangements at a couple of hospitals, and they have worked reasonably well. I also have had a dedicated area within my office, which is a more ideal situation, because patients' progress can be directly monitored, patients get intensive care and education directly from our nurses, and I get to examine patients and monitor their progress each time they come.

Probably one of the more common modes of delivering this therapy has been its administration in the home by one of the many home nursing agencies. In the interests of keeping patients out of the hospital, there has been a marked upsurge in the use of therapies using home nursing services. I have found a wide range of variability both in the skills and the goals of these nursing services and have therefore found wide variability in the kind of care patients with heart failure get in their homes. It makes little sense to me to take some of the patients who have very advanced heart failure and who need to be seen frequently with close monitoring, and place them in a home setting with perhaps the least amount of monitoring. I think many physicians choose this option for patients who have recurrent admissions because they think there is little hope or little else to do for those patients. With rare exceptions, I think that infusion at home is usually not the ideal situation for the end-stage patient. This is very much a point of personal perspective. Many doctors do use these infusions as a sort of end-stage treatment for patients who have not responded to conventional treatments. I personally view them as a temporary situation to help patients over a period of decompensation or to get them onto other, perhaps newer, conventional or investigational drugs. In fact, from the moment I start a patient on an intermittent course of infusions, my goal is to find a way eventually to get him or her off of it. Frequently, when I go to an institution that has been doing infusions for a while, I almost always find patients who have been getting this treatment weekly for as long as two years, or perhaps longer. I generally find that at least half of these patients could easily come off the infusions simply with some adjustments in their medications, and sometimes even with little or no change whatsoever.

Since there has been such a proliferation of home care agencies, I would like to suggest a few criteria for selecting such an agency for a heart failure patient.

1. The agency should have expertise in treating heart disease and heart failure. Several agencies have chosen to concentrate their focus in these areas.
2. The agency should have a cadre of expertly trained nurses who are interested in heart failure. I routinely invite home care nurses to my office so that I can assess the level of knowledge and interest they have, and teach them points I think are important.
3. The agency should have good communications with your doctor. The staff need to be able to transmit lab results, convey anything they notice in the home back to the doctor, and carry out instructions. They must serve as the doctor's eyes and ears.

4. The agency should have definite goals and targets in mind, as should the doctor, to help the patient become more self-reliant and return to a greater level of independence.

POTENTIAL ADVERSE EFFECTS FROM INTERMITTENT INFUSIONS

As I mentioned earlier, there is no clearly proven benefit, in terms of increased survival, for patients who get infusions. Although there has been some suggestion that the use of some of the oral forms of these drugs on a regular basis may actually shorten survival, there has been some inference that intermittent intravenous treatment may also shorten survival; there is no clear proof for that statement either. In fact, I think this is really not a fair comparison. The oral forms were administered in relatively high dosages for chronic periods of time (that is, there was never a period when the patient or heart did not have a high level of drug being exposed to it). With the intermittent infusions, these are usually once weekly, brief exposures to lower dosages of the drugs. Again, these topics are discussed regularly among heart failure experts and the FDA, as well as among patients on the Internet! I hope we will have a more rational approach and understanding in the near future. My experience has been positive in terms of patients feeling better, improved quality of life, and being able to stay out of the hospital. I cannot comment, nor would I expect that patients who need these treatments to necessarily live longer. Perhaps there will be a way to attain that final goal, but for now, I believe that judicious and appropriate use of infusions is beneficial to many.

In order to get these drugs intravenously on a regular basis, patients must either have an intravenous catheter placed each time the treatment is given or have a more permanent form of catheter introduced into the body. The latter is what we call a central line, or a catheter that is usually buried under the skin and inserted into a large vein in the body. There are several kinds of these central line catheters, including Hickman, Groshong, Port-A-Cath, triple lumen, and PICC catheters. All have their advantages and disadvantages, and most require surgical placement. A permanent catheter can be well maintained but increases the risk of infection, which can certainly be a serious problem for a patient who already has heart failure.

There are also risks from the infusion procedure, including an increase in irregular heartbeats because of an increase in the irritability of the heart; large shifts in the electrolytes, that is, in the sodium or potassium in the patient's blood; episodes of low blood pressure; and occasional allergic reactions to the drugs themselves.

In summary, the intermittent infusion of inotropic drugs—when selected judiciously and used in appropriate patients in the appropriate setting for an appropriate interval of time—is a common, useful technique for at least improving the quality of life for many patients with heart failure.

Natrecor (neseritide)

Although I have left the entire section on intravenous infusions pretty much intact, I wanted to be sure to cover what I think is an extremely important advance that may change everything I said.

Earlier I mentioned that a hormone that is normally produced in very small amounts in the heart ventricles can be released in increased amounts when the heart begins to fail; that hormone is B-type natriuretic hormone, or BNP (see the earlier chapter where I discuss using BNP measurement as a test for heart failure). When the heart begins to fail, the ventricles produce even more of this hormone, which is why we can measure it in a blood sample. Well, the reason the heart begins to make more BNP is that this hormone is a naturally occurring way for the body to make the heart work smarter by vasodilating or opening up the arteries and the veins of the body. This BNP hormone also opens up the coronary arteries to supply more blood to the heart itself so it can work better.

Scientists at a company called SCIOS have created this hormone to be used as a medicine and it goes by the name Natrecor, or neseritide. This drug underwent extensive testing and is now available for use for treating patients with heart failure. Most of the time it is used when a patient has retained extra fluid and the body needs some help getting rid of the fluid (I will discuss other uses below). I was fortunate enough to do some of the trials of this medicine before it was released and I really think it is a major advance for treating people when they are hospitalized. This medicine rapidly lowers the pressure or resistance the heart has to work against (which is almost always increased in patients with heart failure). This drug has several other properties but perhaps one of the most important is that unlike the other medications we currently use it does *not* have the tendency to cause extra heartbeats. Natrecor also seems to reverse or lower the levels of some of the bad hormones, which are elevated in heart failure.

One of the trials I helped publish was a study comparing Natrecor to Dobutamine. We saw that on Natrecor, patients needed a shorter period of treatment in the hospital and that once they were discharged they were less likely to be readmitted. Now, this is good news! We also began to see a trend toward decreased survival. Although this observation will require more information and study, it seems like we have a naturally occurring drug that may make a real impact on how patients who are hospitalized for heart failure are treated. Side effects seem to be low. I hope more doctors become familiar with this drug.

Remember that most heart failure patients go to the emergency room when they get very sick. We needed to also find a better way to treat these patients rapidly. Since this drug seems to work quickly and help get the extra salt and fluid out of the body, a group of us have completed a trial (PROACTION) to see whether early administration of Natrecor in the emergency room can keep people out of the hospital or shorten their stay in the hospital. Hopefully, that trial will give us an answer soon.

Naturally, knowing a little about this drug you might think it could be used to help keep patients who are at high risk of being admitted over and over again with heart failure out of the hospital if used in an outpatient area. That study (FUSION) is under way and again I am very hopeful that this will guide us in the near future.

Looking ahead a bit, there is some early scientific evidence that Natrecor might also be able to be given in other ways and perhaps as a subcutaneous injection like insulin. The hopes are that infrequent injections of this medicine may in fact help patients who are very sick and help stabilize them without having to admit them into the hospital. I would hope this would be a treatment that could even be done in your doctor's office. All in all, after all the concerns about the many failings of the intravenous drugs for heart failure, the release of Natrecor seems to be a bright spot on the horizon.

SURGICAL APPROACHES

Another major advance in the last few years has been several remarkable lessons learned about the value of surgical approaches to heart failure. Many doctors and patients share a common misconception that patients who have heart failure "are too sick" to consider a surgical treatment for their heart failure. I think one of the lessons I have learned is that for many patients, unless they do get a surgical treatment they will only get worse and certainly die.

Since the last edition of the book, some of these surgical approaches have changed and some have stayed the same. Obviously, this is a complex topic and cooperation and collaboration are key to a successful strategy. I am truly blessed to work each day with some of the best cardiovascular surgeons I have ever known. The beauty of working with them is that they have the same interest that I do in heart failure and so together we offer a wide range of surgical therapies that most hospitals do not have available. The lesson here is, when a surgical therapy is discussed, try to find a heart failure specialist (or at least a general cardiologist) who has a good collaborative working relationship with a cardiac surgeon. Let me mention a few of the surgical approaches. Some are conventional and other innovative, whereas still others are only investigative.

Coronary Artery Bypass Grafting (or Bypass Surgery)

This is the now common surgery done all over the world. The goal of this surgery is to restore blood flow to the heart muscle to prevent the first or additional heart attacks. What few people know is that studies show that not only should it be considered in patients with normal heart muscle, but in fact, if indicated, it most benefits patients with heart failure or weak heart muscles. Unfortunately, it seems that many surgeons, because of the increased risk, tend to tell patients that the risk is too high—they seem to select patients with only the lowest risk! Again, this is a complex issue, but if you have angina or the doctors confirm that your heart is simply not getting enough blood supply, then restoring this blood supply is critical to not only prevent further worsening of the heart failure but also to possibly reverse some of it!

Mitral Valve Surgery (Mitral Valve Repair or Replacement)

One of the common consequences of heart failure is progressive enlargement of the heart muscle, which causes the heart to stretch and with that stretching pull apart the leaflets of the mitral valve as well as the small papillary muscles that attach to the valve. With this stretching, the mitral valve cannot do its job, which is to prevent leakage of blood backward into the lungs. When this happens, a patient is said to have mitral regurgitation and your doctor can hear this with the stethoscope. An echocardiogram is a better way to assess how much leakage there is.

In some patients, proper medications alone may cause the heart to shrink and lessen or eliminate the mitral regurgitation. However, in many patients the medications alone do not eliminate it and this leakage is responsible for worsening symptoms and progression of the heart failure. Until just a few years ago doctors were taught, however, that if the valve was replaced it would take away the low-pressure relief valve the failing heart had and a patient would not survive this surgery. As the surgeons got smarter they realized they could simply repair the valve using a small ring that went around the mitral valve and pulling it together just the right amount to eliminate the leakage but not interfere with the valves' normal function. The ring is called an annuloplasty ring. Finally, several doctors including Dr. Steve Bolling in Michigan started to repair the mitral valve in patients with weak heart muscles. Instead of them doing poorly, many got remarkably better! Increasingly more and more surgeons are trying this approach. Once again, the presence of a good team including the surgeon and the heart failure specialist are needed to help decide if this is the right option for you.

Cardiac Restraint Devices

Moving ahead, one can imagine that sometimes neither medications nor repairing a mitral valve when it is leaky can prevent the progressive enlargement of the heart. In the last edition I talked about a procedure called dynamic cardiomyoplasty where the back muscle was taken off and wrapped around the heart and them stimulated to contract with the heart. These trials were stopped not because of bad results but simply owing to the amount of surgery required; not enough patients were enrolled into the trials. However, during the period of research we discovered that perhaps more than the effect of the back muscle squeezing the person's heart caused an improvement in the patient. Patients improved by simply having something wrapped around the heart, containing it and preventing it from enlarging even more—this is called cardiac restraint. In fact, one of my patients who had the cardiomyoplasty developed an infection where the pacemaker was and needed it removed. The back muscle, however, remained in place and with the restraint alone he did just as fine.

A series of various cardiac restraint devices have been developed and some are in current trials (the Acorn) and some will begin trials very shortly (the Paracor). They all try to provide support to the heart without interfering with the heart's normal functions of contraction and relaxation. Although all of these devices now have to be put on the heart during a surgical procedure, we are rapidly progressing to finding ways to eventually apply these devices using minimally invasive procedures. In fact, our surgeons are among a select few in the country using a specialized robot to do robotic heart surgery. It is our hope that someday the robotic procedures will allow a more simple and safer way to apply a cardiac restraint device. We are using these devices today in clinical trials to treat either patients with dilated hearts alone or those with dilated hearts and mitral regurgitation. My impressions are that these restraint devices are very helpful in reversing some of the severe enlargement we see—I suspect that these will become a more commonly used treatment and soon we will begin to use them earlier in less ill patients to prevent some of the severe heart enlargement we see today. I think we owe a debt of gratitude to the early investigators who began the experiments with cardiomyoplasty, including Dr. Ray Chiu and Dr. Alain Carpentier.

Left Ventricular Assist Devices

I think many people remember the name Jarvik Heart and recall that it was the first totally artificial heart created by a then young Dr. Robert Jarvik. Well, that form as well as a few variations still exist but are still not commonly used because of the many complications that develop with a large permanent device. One of the lessons we learned was that in most patients, the main problem is with the left ventricle and we soon found that if we could support the left ventricle with a pump that partially or totally took over the left heart function, the patients did pretty well. And so was born a series of left ventricular assist devices (or LVADs).

There are several LVADs on the market but all share some sort of pump that is either contained inside the chest or the abdominal cavity and connected to a power supply to make the pump work. The LVAD we use a lot is the Thoratec LVAD. With this one the pump actually sits outside of the body cavity—this makes it especially useful, since a patient's size alone does not limit his or her ability to get a LVAD. There is a trend to make the power supply implantable as well and that will remain a big challenge since there is limited space inside of the chest.

In the beginning these devices were used only for short periods of time, usually to support the failing heart until a transplant could be done (bridge to transplant). Obviously, these were used only in that select group of patients who were on a heart transplant list. However, as experience grew using these devices for longer periods as a bridge to transplant, two newer concepts emerged. The first was that of using these devices in a more permanent fashion or what we call destination therapy. Recently a large trial called REMATCH showed that compared with medicine treatment alone, patients who got a LVAD survived longer. Unfortunately, these destination therapy patients also eventually died. Many of these deaths stemmed from complications related to having the LVAD in the patient's body permanently.

The final concept has emerged from some early research done by Dr. O. Frasier at the Texas Heart Institute. He observed that patients who had the LVADs as a bridge to transplant had their own heart in pretty good shape at the time of a transplant. People began to wonder if the LVAD could provide a brief vacation or rest period for the heart, after which the heart might then work on its own in an improved fashion; this is called bridge to recovery. Although this concept is still in its early days, we have been extremely successful with this approach when needed and I am amazed at how much even the most weakened heart can recover. Our patients have the LVAD in place between thirty to sixty days and then it is removed. I believe this approach, combined with mitral valve repair when needed and perhaps even with the use of a cardiac restraint device, eventually makes a lot of sense. Stay tuned for more in these areas of research.

External Enhanced Counterpulsation (EECP)

As a transition from talking about surgical procedures to talking about more mundane things like using oxygen, I wanted to say a word about EECP therapy. A long story (but a fascinating one—ask me sometime) made short is that years ago we learned that a large tube placed inside a person's aorta could alter the blood flow to the point of making the heart pumping easier and at the same time improve the feeding of blood back to the heart itself. This is called an intraaortic balloon pump (IABP). Obviously, this has some risks and in fact cannot be used for more than a few days in most cases. A noninvasive way to do the same thing as an IABP was developed and refined and consists of a series of cuffs, like blood pressure cuffs, that go around the outside of the legs and buttocks and then rapidly inflate and deflate, producing the same effects as the IABP but totally noninvasively.

Well, another long story made short, these treatments, given for an hour each day for seven weeks, have been proven to improve the blood flow in the heart and at the same time take away chest pain in patients. Again, by carefully observing these patients it became clear that even patients who had some heart failure benefited and in fact did not seem to get worse. Therefore a large clinical trial of EECP for patients who have heart failure (PEECH trial) is now under way and again I am convinced that this will prove to be a helpful adjunct for the treatment of some patients. Stay tuned here!

Always seeking more options for my patients, I have followed the development of these two surgical procedures for advanced heart failure quite carefully. The Batista procedure has caught many eyes both in the lay and professional press because of its dramatic approach. I have had the pleasure to spend some time with Dr. Randas Batista from Brazil and believe that he truly has performed some excellent procedures, and in fact has quite a bit of rationale behind his procedure. In simple terms, in this procedure a large portion of the weakened and overdilated left ventricle is removed (partial left ventriculectomy). The goal, as he eloquently explains it, is to re-create a more normalized relationship between the mass of the left ventricular tissue and the radius or size of the chamber. Actually, what we try to do medically with drugs such as vasodilators is exactly the same idea—he just does it more radically with a scalpel! Because of the broad interest in this procedure, it is being performed in a few places throughout the world. Because Dr. Batista lacked many resources, his own data are not well scrutinized or summarized. Other places in Brazil and the United States (such as the Cleveland Clinic) are attempting to gather better follow-up information on this procedure. In the few published reports, many of which are quite early as of this writing, there seem to be some patients who clearly benefit, whereas for others the procedure is not successful or only partially successful for a relatively short duration. A major problem currently is trying to predict or select those patients who *will* benefit over the long haul. I believe we will know more about this exciting and scientifically interesting approach over the next one to two years.

An important part of Dr. Batista's procedure has been to repair the leaky and enlarged mitral valve. This has caused some interest in the possibility that the mitral valve operation alone, by decreasing the leakage of blood back through the mitral valve, may play a major role in the improvement in many patients. Other surgeons, such as Dr. Steve Bolling, employ this approach almost exclusively. Therefore, there are many different approaches in between what I call the Batista-like operations. The problem with all of this is that it makes it difficult to compare results when precisely the same operation is not being performed by everyone.

SUPPLEMENTAL OXYGEN

One of the most frequent questions I hear from patients and their families is whether the patient with heart failure should have an oxygen supply in the home. This usually involves a two-part answer. Since the weak heart and congested lungs frequently have a difficult time getting enough oxygen into the blood circulation or delivering enough oxygen to the rest of the body, it seems logical that supplementing the oxygen supply would make the patient feel better. In fact, this is true, and it's one of the first treatments we frequently give when we treat patients in the hospital. Moreover, oxygen can be considered a drug in that it has important effects in opening up the arteries and lowering pressure within the lungs.

On the other hand, I have all too frequently seen patients with heart failure who are slowly getting worse over a period of days or weeks take to using their home oxygen on a regular basis, only to appear in the emergency room with severe heart failure. I think a false reliance on oxygen as a means of feeling better for the short term often backfires: It lets the patient get progressively sicker before calling the doctor and often results in a longer hospital stay. I have even seen patients rely on using their oxygen at home to such an extent that they limit their exercise because they are tethered to the oxygen cord.

Your doctor can do certain tests to help decide whether oxygen will be helpful for you to use in your home. You should be aware that Medicare has very stringent criteria for those who qualify for home oxygen, and if you do not meet these qualifications, you may end up paying a hefty bill for oxygen use in your home.

ELASTIC SUPPORT STOCKINGS

Many patients who have had bypass surgery are given a pair of white elastic stockings to wear after their surgery. These stockings may prevent blood clots from forming in the legs while a person is immobile and act as a mechanical means of stimulating the blood return from the legs back to the heart. A similar situation applies to patients with heart failure, many of whom also have a great many "varicose veins." In fact, much of the cause for the varicose vein formation is due to the failing heart and very high pressures that impair the blood return to the heart from the legs.

The elastic stockings can certainly provide a great deal of comfort and support for patients who have leg edema. These stockings should usually reach above the knee, because the lower ones can constrict the return of fluid at the knee and may not eliminate the swelling of the legs. There are various kinds of elastic stockings available, but usually, staff at your hospital, pharmacy, or hospital supply company can recommend a good brand for you. Usually, the white ones you get in the hospital after surgery are really just antiembolism stockings—to prevent blood clots from forming. True anticompression stockings are different and offer more resistance, particularly when you are standing up. You can discuss this with your doctor or, better yet, with local hospital supply store staff. These usually need to be fitted properly to provide the most benefit.

Since leg swelling tends to diminish at night, when people are lying flat, it is generally best to put these stockings on the first thing in the morning. If they are fitted properly, they should not be difficult to get on; however, the process may represent a good deal of effort for the patient with heart failure, and often the help of a spouse or other relative is needed. As the swelling in the legs subsides, the stockings may become loose, in which case patients may want either to go without them or get a better-fitting pair. If more swelling develops in the legs, the stockings may become uncomfortable and should then be avoided.

I have certainly found that support stockings are an important adjunct for many patients who continue to have lower leg swelling, and they are often a worthwhile investment for my patients.

13

Quality of Life

On the occasion of his ninetieth birthday party, Senator Strom Thurmond of South Carolina had many people express the wish that they hoped to be able to attend his hundredth birthday party. He said to them that if they ate the proper diet and exercised, they might be able to be there!

—NATIONAL PUBLIC RADIO

Two years ago, I couldn't make a piece of toast; last Sunday, I cooked dinner for sixteen.

—PATIENT A. P.

PATIENT R. P. (AGE SEVENTY-THREE): *Hey, Doc, I want to be able to go to my granddaughter's wedding.*
DR. SILVER: *Oh, when is that?*
PATIENT R. P.: *Eighteen years from now.*

The Golden Years? What's that? It seems someone forgot the G.

—A PATIENT'S SPOUSE

In treating patients with heart failure, there are obviously many goals, not just increased longevity. Since patients with heart failure are limited in their activity because of shortness of breath and fatigue, an additional goal would be to ameliorate these symptoms. Another goal is to improve the patient's quality of life. I must say that this is not a topic to which I pay mere lip service but it is, in fact, one of the primary goals I have in mind for each and every one of my patients. It is clear that the overall quality of life for those patients whose heart failure is so advanced and who have suffered for so long is not going to change significantly regardless of the treatment we could offer them. This is particularly true for the elderly patient with heart failure. Also, there are limited treatments to make the most sick patients feel completely well again, and therefore the focus really must be on quality of life.

One of the problems that arises when we address the subject of quality of life is, of course, how to define it and, even more difficult, how to measure it. In recent years, there have been some major advances toward trying to quantify or measure the quality of life for patients with heart failure. This has been extremely important, for we can now, finally, evaluate how the various treatments we try for our patients with heart failure affect not only what we doctors call "end points," such as death or hospitalization, but also the quality of a patient's life. Thanks to people such as Drs. Thomas Rector and Jay Cohn at the University of Minnesota, the Living with Heart Failure Questionnaire (that follows) has been developed and rigorously tested to show that it really is a valid instrument for measuring the quality of life in patients with heart failure. As you can see from the questions, this questionnaire touches on many of the common limitations patients with heart failure have and gives us good insight into both the physical and the emotional, or psychological, component of a patient's heart failure.

LIVING WITH HEART FAILURE QUESTIONNAIRE[1]

[1]Copyright University of Minnesota, 1986. Reprinted with permission of Dr. Thomas Rector.

Did your heart failure prevent you from living as you wanted during the last month by:

1. causing swelling in your ankles?
2. making working around the house or yard difficult?
3. making relating to or doing things with your friends or family difficult?
4. making you sit or lie down to rest during the day?
5. making you tired, fatigued, or low on energy?
6. making working to earn a living difficult?
7. making walking about or climbing stairs difficult?
8. making you short of breath?
9. making sleeping well at night difficult?
10. making you eat less of the foods you like?
11. making going places away from home difficult?
12. making sexual activities difficult?
13. making recreational pastimes, sports, or hobbies difficult?

14. making it difficult for you to concentrate or remember things?
15. giving you side effects from medications?
16. making you worry?
17. making you feel depressed?
18. costing you money for medical care?
19. making you feel a loss of self-control?
20. making you stay in a hospital?
21. making you feel you are a burden to your family or friends?

Many years ago, before such questionnaires were used for patients with heart failure, I asked a group of my patients who had been in a drug trial and had received an experimental medication to fill out a form with some questions on it, namely, how they learned about their heart failure, which sources of information were helpful, and how they felt about being asked to join a drug study. I also surveyed them on their knowledge of the other treatments that were available. Many of the patients indicated that they now knew quite a bit about their heart failure; had learned primarily from talking with physicians, staff, and other patients; felt privileged to participate in a drug trial and felt they had received special care because of their participation; and so on. At the end of the questionnaire, I left an open space, inviting patients to indicate anything else they thought I should know about them or about how their heart failure had affected their lives. One man in his forties, who had heart failure for some time before he came to see me, wrote, "Not hardly anything except no work, no sex, no beer, and no money!" This would have amounted to a poor score on any quality-of-life questionnaire, and it certainly made an impression on me. I have never forgotten that if I haven't improved a person's quality of life, I haven't treated that person completely.

There are various other measurement tools available to assess a patient's quality of life, including the Heart Failure Functional Status Inventory, the Multiple Affect Adjective List, the Psychosocial Adaptation to Illness Scale, and the Short Forms 12 and 36 (SF 12 and SF 36), to name a few. It is interesting to note that some of the objective measurements we make on a patient with heart failure, such as ejection fraction, very commonly bear little correlation to quality-of-life measurements. And probably an even more important observation is the conclusion from a recent study, namely, that the patient's baseline quality of life correlated significantly with overall longevity. Now you might say that this reflects the fact that the patients who felt better initially were the ones who lived longer, but I think this could also be interpreted to reflect the notion that patients with a better mental attitude and quality of life do better and survive longer despite an initial poor functional status. As Dr. Bernie Siegel says in *Love, Medicine, and Miracles* (New York: HarperCollins), "Exceptional patients have the ability to throw statistics aside—to say, 'I can be a survivor'—even when the doctor isn't wise enough to do so."

Look again at the third quotation at the beginning of this chapter. It was from a seventy-three-year-old gentleman whom I was seeing for the first time. He was very sick with heart failure and, in fact, had quite limited physical capacity. He had just been discharged from a long hospitalization and was coming to my office to see if he could find a way to improve his heart failure and stay out of the hospital. It was at the end of my conversation with him that he made clear to me his goal of going to his granddaughter's wedding. I fell for his joke, but I am happy to report that he is today doing well and that now his granddaughter's wedding is only thirteen years away!

I mention this story because on the very same day, I saw another gentleman with equally severe heart failure. This gentleman was coming to me from another cardiologist to see what we could offer him for his advanced heart failure. I gave him almost exactly the same options I gave the first patient, and he said he would consider them all and get back to me within the next couple of days. I was deeply disturbed late that evening to get a phone call from an emergency room reporting that this patient had been admitted with a self-inflicted gunshot wound. I found out later that this man had a rather long history of depression and that this was not his first suicide attempt. However, I think these two cases suggest that these two patients, despite equal severity of disease, felt quite differently about the quality of their life and viewed the same options differently—so differently that their views affected their approaches to getting more help. So even initial quality of life may influence how a patient accepts and responds to the idea of treatment for heart failure.

It is always one of my goals to try to assess the patient's quality of life from the very outset and to try to make major changes in his or her quality of life even prior to attempting to make major improvements in his or her functional status. A recent study found that up to 43 percent of patients with advanced heart failure had feelings of depression, hostility, and anger because of their limited daily activity. We often find that simple changes make big differences in the quality of life and help motivate people to stick with their treatments. An example of this is simply changing the second diuretic dose to about four in the afternoon rather than nine or ten at night, thus allowing people to get a little bit more sleep at night. Other simple things—showing patients how they can eat flavorful meals while restricting the salt in their diet, allowing them to drive again, encouraging them to begin some low-level exercise—are also important in improving quality of life.

Finally, let me say that this whole issue of quality of life, despite the development of better tools to measure it, remains extremely complex. Certainly, the quality of life of the patient who suffers with heart failure needs to be addressed, but I think, in a broader sense, quality of life refers to the patient in the context of family and friends. For example, I have one patient who seems to be honest when he says that he feels his quality of life has improved and that he feels well most of the time these days. Unfortunately, when I talk to members of his family, who are so doting and meticulous in caring for him, I get the idea that although the patient feels well, the quality of life for his family has not improved! In fact, I think that their quality of life is worse because of all the things to which we have taught them to pay attention. I think this all comes down to a need for having good communication among the patient, the family, the doctor, and the doctor's staff—communication in all directions, which sometimes involves specific, open-ended discussions about what is important to the patient and to the family, and how to find a happy medium for everyone. I remember one near-battle in my office when a patient came in with his wife. I had only met the wife on a couple of occasions, and she had very little to say. At the end of our visit, the patient said to me, "Doc, please tell her that I can have some cheese." When this man first became my patient, my staff and I examined his eating habits and found that he was eating a great deal of salt in his food. We told him to limit certain high-salt foods such as cheese, which he tried to do. A few weeks later, he reported, "Doc, I've really cut down on virtually everything, but the one thing I really must have is some cheese." From the passion in this man's eyes, it was clear that allowing him to eat a little cheese on a rare occasion would make his quality of life better and the rest of his low-salt diet much more palatable. The problem, however, was that his wife, who had never heard me relax my taboo against cheese, felt that she needed to be the self-appointed "salt police" for the patient. Husband and wife battled back and forth until I intervened. I tried to make clear to the wife how much I appreciated her efforts, how I wished that she could be in the home of many of my other patients who needed to be reminded to stick to their diet, and, finally, how I was reducing the severity of my injunction against cheese in her husband's case and allowing him to have a little at his own discretion. Although the issue surrounding food would seem to be a minor one, in this family, at least, this simple solution seemed to make a great deal of difference in determining the quality of life in the long run, not only for this gentleman but for his entire family.

Improving the quality of life is an extremely important ingredient in the entire treatment regimen for patients with heart failure. I emphasize again the importance of communicating this issue to the physician, because almost always, some happy medium can be worked out to help improve the quality of life for patients and their families.

14

How to Stay
Out of the Hospital

Here are the facts. The average patient with heart failure has 1.7 hospital admissions per year. The worse your heart failure, the more often you end up in the hospital. Also, the worse your care, often, the more times you end up in the hospital. Drugs, diet, exercise, and positive emotions can all impact this reality, but hospitalization is often part of the reality for most patients. I have found great benefit, especially when teaching young doctors about heart failure, to keep in mind several things when a patient is hospitalized for heart failure. Focus on the main problems for the admission; in other words, don't try and fix everything in the hospital—this is not the environment to fix it all. Also, I tell them to take advantage of the hospitalization to help the patient find ways to *not* be hospitalized again! This is usually a process of education. Therefore, in the first edition, I wrote this chapter because no matter what stage people with heart failure are in, everyone wants to stay out of the hospital. Many patients have told me of its value to them and so I have updated it for this book.

A lot of people first find out about their heart failure when they are initially admitted to a hospital, and of course, any further admissions to the hospital represent a lack of progress, a sign of illness, and a step backward. It is common to have multiple admissions, and as the heart failure progresses, the time away from the hospital frequently becomes shorter and shorter. Perhaps you're one of those people who are told they have heart failure in their doctor's office, and you've not yet been hospitalized. Staying out of the hospital is one of your primary goals—and indeed, it should be. Or you may be a family member for whom the hospitalization of a loved one is causing difficulty—the emotional pain in seeing your relative hospitalized, the inconvenience for you in getting back and forth to the hospital, the need to rearrange schedules, and the disruption of your everyday routine. There are many more reasons why we don't like to see patients with heart failure hospitalized, including the large economic burden, the time away from work, and the sense of illness that hospitals provide.

You may be a hospital administrator or a politician concerned with rising health care costs, who realizes that for people over the age of sixty-five, heart failure is the number one cause of admissions to all hospitals across our country. From an administrator's point of view, you are aware that with every hospitalization for a senior citizen with heart failure, you lose money. For example, currently Medicare reimburses a hospital just a little over $3,700 for every heart failure admission to the hospital and expects a length of stay in the hospital of no more than three or four days. However, the facts are that the average length of stay for a heart failure admission may be more than seven or eight days, and the hospital cost, including room, medications, X rays, blood tests, intravenous solutions, and so forth can amount to well over $10,000. If you were in business and losing approximately $6,000 on your number one sales item, you would be broke in no time! That is why some of the effort to do a better job with heart failure has been motivated by our cost-conscious side of the health care system.

It is clear that staying out of the hospital once you have heart failure is a measure of success. It represents the success of your treatment, it represents your ability to control your heart failure symptoms and progression by limiting your fluid and your salt, and in many respects, it reflects the success in communication between you, your family, your physician, and other heart failure professionals. I hope that when you are in the hospital, a major "tune-up" will be performed so that all the extra fluid retained in your body that causes the swelling in your legs and in your liver, the fluid in your lungs, and so on, is removed and you get down to your dry weight. Also, you will have the opportunity to review the importance of fluid and salt restriction with one of the nurses, the doctor, or the dietitian. New medications may be prescribed, and you will have a chance to become familiar with their effects and regimen. Perhaps an exercise program will be discussed with you during that hospital period, or perhaps new support systems will be established for you as you talk with other heart failure patients, learn about support groups, or arrange to have visiting home health services after your discharge.

STEPS TO TAKE AFTER DISCHARGE

Whatever steps are taken in the hospital, it is imperative that you maximize those steps once you become an outpatient. What I would like to do in this chapter is list some of the important steps that you should take immediately upon being discharged from the hospital in order to prevent another admission. If you have never been hospitalized, these are steps that may help prevent an admission.

Check Your Weight

Surprisingly, body weight is one of the most informative and accurate measurements doctors and nurses use to help monitor patients with heart failure. In the hospital, patients are weighed on a daily basis, primarily to see if the extra fluid is coming off at a proper rate. Yes, there are other ways to assess fluid retention—by examining the legs, listening to the lungs, monitoring what doctors and nurses call "I and O," or fluid intake and output—but measuring a patient's weight is really a simple procedure that is reproducible from day to day.

Therefore, one of the most important pieces of medical equipment you can have in your home is a good scale. You do not need to purchase an expensive doctor's office–type scale; any scale, whether digital or spring, will do. The main idea is to get into the habit of taking your weight each day at the same time, with the same amount of clothing on.

Many patients weigh themselves first thing in the morning. You should probably urinate first and then weigh yourself; do this either before or after your bath or shower, but preferably before you eat your breakfast and with approximately the same amount of clothing on (or even in the nude). At least for the first few weeks, or until you are well in the habit of noting it each day, you should write your weight down on a piece of paper. A written record that shows the trend in your weight over a period of time will be helpful when you call your doctor or go in for an office visit.

Our nurses are always catching patients who have been told to weigh themselves but don't. Invariably, a patient will call and report being a little bit more short of breath since an office visit three weeks earlier. The nurse's first question will be, "Well, what is your weight today?" so that it can be compared to the weight taken three weeks ago. Patients who weigh themselves regularly can provide that piece of information immediately and precisely, whereas those who have been skipping their daily chore of checking their weight will usually say, "Oh, it's about the same" or "It's up just a little" or "I've noticed my clothes are a little bit tighter." But that kind of subjective measurement just won't do. You need to check your weight on a daily basis.

Monitor Your Fluid Intake and Urinary Output

Measurements of fluid intake and output are used in the hospital to make sure that a limited amount of fluid goes into the heart failure patient each day and that a sufficient amount of urine is being produced each day. When we are trying to get fluid off a patient, we want the output to exceed the intake. Once there is a period of stability, the intake and output more closely coincide, though usually the output still exceeds the input by a slight amount. That is because in addition to the fluids taken in, the body produces water as part of its natural metabolism.

Monitoring your intake at home is a fairly simple job. There are a variety of techniques people have used, but none is as simple as filling a 1.5-quart container with water and pouring an equivalent amount of this water out every time you take some liquid to drink. When the container is empty, you are done with your fluids for the day. This is a particularly good thing to do in the first weeks after you get home from the hospital, until you can accurately gauge exactly how much fluid is included in your fluid restriction. People often say, "Oh, Doc, I'm not drinking that much" or "I really don't take in that much pop or juice or milk each day," but once they start to keep track, they find out that they are in fact consuming a great deal of fluid.

The same sort of idea applies to output. Many people take home from the hospital the measuring cups or urinals they used there to keep track of their daily urinary output. This can be a little harder to do than it was during the hospital stay, particularly if a person is active and spends a great deal of time away from home. That's why measuring the weight is the most simple and efficient way to keep track of the fluid status of your body. However, many patients do keep quite accurate track of their urinary output, and I have had more than one patient report daily urine output to me with an accuracy of one cubic centimeter. Again, once there has been a period of stability and you are familiar with how much urine output you're having on a daily basis, you do not have to keep track of this as much, unless instructed to do so by your doctor.

After a few weeks of measuring output, people are actually quite good at estimating how much urine they produce on a daily basis and can quickly tell you if their urinary output has dropped slightly, which is often one of the first signs that fluid retention is going on and that an oral diuretic has lost its effect. You should be aware that one of the common reasons for people with heart failure ending up back in the hospital is indiscretion in dietary habits, particularly in fluid or salt intake. Therefore, monitoring these "I's and O's" is really quite important.

Monitoring Your Sodium Intake

Since indiscretion in the diet is a common reason for another bout of heart failure, we urge people to become familiar with the total sodium contained in a 2,000-milligram sodium chloride diet, although most people use avoidance of salt as the basic way to monitor their sodium restriction. However, many patients do keep accurate records of their sodium intake and can tell you how many grams of salt they consume each day.

Quite often, it is the spouse of the heart failure patient who keeps track of, and close control over, the sodium intake. I recall one patient in particular who came to see me after hospitalization for heart failure. His wife brought in some of the most meticulous records I have ever seen. They included every cubic centimeter of fluid taken in and every drop of urine put out. In fact, every morsel of food that went into this gentleman's body had a sodium content estimated and entered into a large handbook the couple carried around with them. The sections were color coded and divided into three periods of the day—overall, a splendid piece of work. For a short time, the gentleman did well, and then I began to notice some fluid accumulation. A quick check of the records showed that something was amiss. After I spoke to the husband alone, I learned that he considered his wife to be so meticulous and so controlling in monitoring him that as a form of rebellion, he was managing to sneak by the local hot dog stand on a daily basis. The point here is that you really do need to restrict your intake of fluid and salt, and that conscientious behavior is usually well reflected in your body weight; close counts of salt and fluid intake are primarily for educational purposes, that is, to train you to recognize what a proper heart failure diet is.

Know Your Medicines and Have an Ample Supply

Commonly, during a hospital visit for heart failure, various new medicines are started, and those a patient has been on for a long time are adjusted. One of my pet peeves is that most of the discharge planning, or preparation of the patient to go home from the hospital, takes place about five minutes before the patient walks out the door. It usually takes place right in the middle of the period when the nurse is terribly busy with other patients. The fact that the patient is eager to get out of the hospital and a family member has just come on a lunch break and is eager to get the patient home provides an added sense of pressure and urgency. Usually, patients are given a scrap of paper with so-called discharge instructions and sent on their merry way.

Ideally, the discharge planning process should start when the person is first admitted to the hospital. During hospitalization, new medications patients are receiving should be explained and shown to them, so that they can begin to recognize the form of the medication. We strongly recommend and try to use a medication chart that not only lists each medication along with the dose being prescribed but also indicates what the medication is for and at what time it should be taken. Therefore, to further your goal of staying out of the hospital, you need to know exactly what your medications are and precisely when to take them. There are many other things you need to know about your medications, such as whether they should be taken with food or without, whether they should be taken with other medicines or not, and what you should do if you miss a dose by an hour or so (some medications should be taken anyway, and others should be avoided because they would come too close to the next dose).

These are questions that should be addressed to your doctor or nurse, but sometimes a pharmacist can give plenty of good information.

Another point I'd like to make is that patients should, whenever possible, become totally familiar with their medications and even carry a medication list with them at all times. I have seen a wide variety of these, from computer-generated printouts to handwritten lists, but they all work as long as the patients themselves know their medications. Many patients have their spouse or caregiver or home health nurse prepare their medications. This can often be a disaster, because if that person is unavailable, some patients no longer know which medications to take, and a few simple medication errors can land them right back in the hospital. You will also notice that when you go to your doctor's office for a visit, he or she may change medications based on your progress; you should have a way of quickly and clearly updating your medication list, so that when you arrive home from the doctor's office, there will be no confusion about exactly what changes were made.

Just as bad as not knowing your medicines or not knowing when to take them is running out of them. A large percentage of the phone calls doctors get on weekends are for prescription refills. When I see a patient in the office, one of the last questions I almost always ask is, "Do you have enough of your medicines?" Many people do know, but it's surprising how many are not aware of the supply they have on hand. In fact, we are seeing more problems with this as more and more people are using mail-in prescription services. These services usually supply a one-month or a three-month supply of medication at one time. However, if at the end of one month we double the dose of a certain medication, a person will run out of that medication before the next prescription is due to be mailed to them. Therefore, it is always a good idea to check the medicines to make sure you have an ample supply. If there is ever a question about whether you are going to continue on a certain medication, that is, if your doctor has indicated to you that he or she might be eliminating a particular drug in the future or changing to a different formulation, check with your doctor's office before you refill that prescription; I hate to see a person buy a fresh supply of an expensive medication just before I discontinue prescribing it.

Know How Much Activity Is Expected of You

A great deal of confusion arises regarding how much activity patients should have once they go home from the hospital. I believe doctors always expect that patients will be more active at home, yet it is common for patients and family members to believe that patients should maintain the same activity level they had in the hospital. Lack of communication on this point frequently leads to patients remaining quite inactive at home, which is a problem not only because it results in a deconditioning of their muscles, but also because it takes away one of the important tools doctors have in assessing how patients are progressing. For example, if you limit yourself to staying indoors and walking from room to room, your activity is so little that your doctor does not know how much activity you are really capable of.

You should ask, and your doctor should tell you, exactly what activities you may pursue once you leave the hospital (or once you are diagnosed). If this was not mentioned at the outset and you are limiting your activity to the point that you feel you could certainly do a great deal more, do not hesitate to call and discuss this with your doctor; he or she may not realize how limited your activity is. I recall seeing a particular patient intermittently for a couple of months as an outpatient. She was doing fairly well, and I wanted to cut back on some of the treatments she was getting. I asked her if she got out of breath when she exerted herself, and she replied "no." I asked her if she got fatigued with her daily activities, and again she replied "no." It was not until I specifically asked her what her daily activities were that she replied, "Well, doctor, you know that I never take more than twenty steps at a time." She then proceeded to explain to me that two years earlier, when she left the hospital after becoming ill for the first time, her doctor at the time told her never to take more than twenty steps at any one time. She had followed these instructions to a T and for the subsequent two years had severely limited her activity.

You should get a clear picture about what your level of activity is and what you can and cannot do. I commonly tell patients progressively to do more and to try things. I tell them that when they get tired or feel exhausted or get out of breath, these are simply the ways the body uses to tell them that they've reached their limit for the moment. I encourage them to go back and try the same activity the next day or the day after to see if they can't do it a bit better or a little longer. Also, I often tell patients to do what they can or gradually to begin a very slow walking program at least until I see them in the office and perform a cardiopulmonary exercise test. Once I do that exercise test, I can frequently tell a patient more precisely what he or she should be doing and at what heart rate and, in fact, whether more exercise is going to help or hurt.

Keep an Accurate Assessment of Your Symptoms

Dr. Bernie Siegel has written another wonderful book, *How to Live Between Office Visits* (New York: HarperCollins). Although the book primarily promotes patient empowerment, faith, belief, and emotions, the practical question for the heart failure patient still remains: What should you do between office visits? Obviously, if there is a marked worsening of your symptoms after you leave the hospital or doctor's office, this is something about which you need to call your doctor. However, you also need to keep track of minor changes, the day-to-day changes that are so important in helping your doctor guide your progress. For example, I frequently tell patients that I am changing their medication but want them to pay particular attention to what their energy level is like by noting such things as whether they are able to make their bed in the morning with less effort, whether they take fewer naps during the day, and whether they feel less fatigued at the end of the day. It is this sensitivity to changes in your body and in the way you feel that is so important in monitoring your progress—and, by the same token, in monitoring any changes in the other direction. Feeling more fatigued during the day, taking more naps, having more difficulty sleeping, discovering that doing a chore you've been used to doing on a regular basis is now more difficult—any of these can be an early sign that you need more help for your heart failure.

In fact, it is usually these early, subtle changes (like being able to walk up a flight of stairs without having to stop in the middle or at the top) that indicate when the medicines are finally kicking in and progress is being made. Therefore, you can help keep yourself out of the hospital by keeping accurate track of these common, day-to-day activities. You should also know when to call your doctor. You will usually be given some guidelines; you may be instructed to call if, for example, your weight goes up by a certain amount, if you experience more shortness of breath, if you notice more swelling in your legs, if you have more difficulty breathing, and so on. If there is ever a question as to whether you should call your doctor, you probably should call. If you feel uncomfortable about a certain situation or feeling, a quick call is usually easier to deal with and will be more satisfying to both you and your doctor than an emergency hospital visit at two in the morning.

Having a practice that is dedicated exclusively to taking care of very sick patients with heart failure, I am honestly amazed at how few of my patients end up in the emergency room or hospitalized, or even how few calls I get on the weekend. I attribute this mostly to the wonderful education the patients get from the nurses but also to the encouragement we give our patients to call during the week to try to clarify little problems before they become big ones. Therefore, good communication is one of the factors that will keep you out of the hospital.

Do All Those Little Things You Learned in the Hospital

Do the little things you learned during your hospital stay, even if you think they're not important, and even if you don't like doing them because they remind you of being hospitalized. For example, when people come into the hospital with swollen legs, I usually order a pair of the thigh-high support hose and have the nurses help the patient put them on each morning and take them off at bedtime. These are yours, but most people take that souvenir of the hospital and neatly pack it away in one of their drawers. I encourage patients to use these stockings, particularly when their legs are swollen, but even when there is no swelling, the stockings provide a good deal of support and help the blood flow return in the legs. The legs of heart failure patients are clearly not normal and have altered patterns of blood flow return. If they are prescribed for you, you should try to use these stockings. You may have been given a lot of literature regarding heart failure in the hospital or in the doctor's office; you should review this information periodically and see if you can't learn one more thing about your heart failure each time you read through the materials.

If you can find a heart failure support group in your area, or you've been contacted by Mended Hearts or another support service, try to get involved. I think this gives patients a good frame of reference, allowing them to see what other patients do under similar circumstances, to compare notes, and to feel more like a member of a community and less like an isolated person with a disease.

Soon after the first edition of *Success with Heart Failure* was published, my publisher sent me another interesting book published by his company called *Take Charge of Your Hospital Stay.* (Perseus Publishing) Written by Karen Keating McCann, an exceptional health writer, this book left me with my eyes opened! She presents the hard-hitting but realistic problems surrounding the decision to be admitted to a hospital and covers many topics effectively, including finding a "care partner" or liaison, checking your medication and tests, inquiring about rehabilitation services and nursing homes, and wrestling with your hospital bills. Although some of the issues are not directly related to patients with heart failure, this hard-hitting book is the patient's friend and a terrific resource any time a hospitalization is needed—and unfortunately, for most patients it will be. The trick, then, is to find ways to make the hospital visit be of benefit with the least risk—the old risk-benefit ratio!

Use Your Home Health Services

Many people go home from the hospital with some home nursing personnel, including visiting nurses, physical therapists, home health aides, and homemakers. You should know precisely who these people are and what their functions are when they come to your home. Also, you should know which doctor ordered their services and to whom they are reporting. You can use them as a liaison for many of your questions, although my experience has been that although they generally provide good general nursing care, most home care companies do not provide specific information for heart failure patients. That is changing, however, and some specialized companies are emerging that are dedicated to providing general cardiac services and are quite knowledgeable about heart failure care.

If a physical therapist comes to your home, your job is to work hard with that therapist for the duration of the visit, not to entertain the person socially. The same thing is true for the home health nurse. These people are usually kind and compassionate, but their job is to find out how you are doing, and your job is to find out what other information you need to know about your heart failure. You need to use these professionals for the resources they are. They can also be important stopgaps to help you avoid returning to the hospital. If you are experiencing symptoms—more shortness of breath, more leg swelling, an increase in weight—you may be able to get a home health nurse to come to your home that evening or the next day with instructions from the doctor before you would be able to reach the doctor yourself. Also, the nurse might be better able to assess your symptoms than you and can help you decide whether you need to go to the emergency room or whether you can wait to contact a doctor the following morning.

Educate Yourself

Once you are home from the hospital, besides doing all the things your doctors and nurses ask you to do, you should take it upon yourself to find out more about your condition and what can be done for it. This includes not only going to the library to read some general information about heart disease but also perhaps visiting a medical library, getting information from your local heart association, and keeping your eyes and ears open for radio and television broadcasts about advances in the treatment of heart failure. I am not surprised when we get a half-dozen phone calls the day after a news broadcast about some advance in the treatment of heart failure, all inquiring about that new technique or new investigational drug. What actually does surprise me is that we only receive a half-dozen calls. Extrapolating from my experience, I conclude that of the thousands and thousands of people who heard that announcement, most have not yet begun to take full charge and control of their disease. It can be argued that in the hospital patients lose a lot of their privacy and power—and although there are many ways to combat this, the truth is that the hospital environment is far from ideal, from both the physician's and the patient's standpoint—but once a patient is out of the hospital and becomes his or her own person again, it is their duty to regain empowerment and take control of the disease. In other words, at that point the professionals are not the patients' masters or leaders but simply their guides.

During the week or so after hospitalization you should reread the materials you were given, rethink the things you were told, and try to make a sensible plan that fits with your lifestyle and your goals. If things do not fit, discussing them with your doctor at the next visit is probably one of the most important parts of that visit.

I believe the steps outlined here will be helpful to you as you try to plan your own course of therapy after you've left the hospital (and will certainly help you avoid an initial hospitalization). I think they focus on areas in which you can take control and in many ways be the master of your fate in terms of preventing a hospital visit.

The wife of one of my patients said to me recently that she and her husband felt there were not many positive things going on in his life. He had to watch his fluid and salt intake, but only the exercise I recommended for him felt to him like something he could control. I feel that all the steps I've presented so far in this chapter—watching fluid intake, watching salt consumption, exercising, taking your daily weight—are things that you can actively become involved in and really make a significant difference in the overall progress and outcome of your heart failure.

HOW TO VISIT YOUR DOCTOR

The next step after you have been out of the hospital is planning for your next (or your initial) outpatient visit with your doctor. Often, patients don't know what to bring with them to the visit in terms of records, and I thought I would suggest a few things that might make your visit more efficient and more informative.

If you have been keeping accurate track of your daily weights (as you should) and have monitored your intake and output, bring those records with you. What happens to your weight in your first two or three days at home is often much more important to me than the differences between your weight at the hospital before you left and your weight in my office on the day of your visit; your home scale will be the most consistent over those initial few days.

You should also bring with you all of your medication bottles, as well as your list of medications. Actually, one thing that really bothers me is that in the hospital, often university centers where interns and residents work, patients go home with a new set of prescriptions that are often similar but not the same brands as the pills they have at home. Often, some changes are made in the hospital to try to improve patients but little attempt is made by the resident or intern to reestablish patients back onto the pills they were taking when they came into the hospital. And these doctors have little knowledge or concern that patients may have just spent $75 for their prescription for Vasotec, only to be discharged with a new $75 prescription for another, similar medication. Therefore, even before discharge, review all your medications with the hospital staff and make sure that the new medications are not similar to the ones you have at home!

At your first visit, the doctor or nurses will check that the prescriptions you actually got filled are exactly what the doctor wants you to take. Yes, it is possible for doctors to make errors in writing prescriptions and for pharmacists to make errors in filling them. So on the first hospital discharge visit, I make sure that the medication list is accurate and that the identity and dosage of a patient's pills reflect what I think they are taking. You should also bring with you any other medications the doctor may not know you are taking, including vitamins, minerals, or over-the-counter medications. You may think these medications are safe, but they may have important interactions with the drugs you are taking. Bringing them in gives the doctor a good opportunity to review that possibility with you. You should also be prepared to tell the doctor what activities you have been engaging in since you left the hospital. I always find helpful the remarks patients make regarding what they think they are able to do, whether they get more or less winded than before, and whether they feel more or less fatigued after a particular activity. I also ask patients what they do on a daily basis. If they have not thought about this or have not written down a few notes, they usually can't tell me what their activities have been. I am particularly interested in what they are able to do when they leave the house, for example, if they are able to walk around the mall, visit their children, or go out for dinner with friends and family. At this office visit, I welcome questions regarding fluid and salt restriction, and though we do not solicit them, it is surprising how often we get true confessions about failing to stick to the dietary restrictions, along with fervent promises to reform.

At every office visit you should bring a list of questions you have regarding your condition and treatment. Now, not every health care question needs to be addressed or is appropriate for the doctor who treats your heart failure. For example, when patients come to see me for their heart failure and they have another primary care doctor, I'm usually not the one to answer questions about their diabetes, although I will inquire about it. Also, if they have another medical problem unrelated to their heart failure, I usually will refer that to their primary care physician. Often, however, patients don't know which doctor they should address which question to, and it is fair game to bring them up.

The questions patients often ask at the first office visit have to do with their recent hospitalization; most want to know the nature and meaning of the results of all the testing that was done in the hospital. They might also begin to ask questions about what the alternatives for therapy are and what the plans are for their short-, medium-, and long-term care. Commonly, questions come up regarding their ability to drive again or to travel. I often feel that patients and their families believe the cardiologist is the only person capable of deciding when the patient can drive. For those who have severe irregularities of the heartbeat, the answer is clear: Patients who have suffered a sudden passing out because of the irregularity of their heartbeats or who have implanted defibrillators should not drive. However, many people with heart failure do not have these problems, and the question always arises (usually from adult children concerned about a parent) as to whether they are capable of driving. Patients often reason that since they have been driving safely for many years, they can continue to do so. They usually add that they are not going to go far, only within the neighborhood. At this point, one of my nurses always hastens to add the fact that most accidents occur within a mile of home.

The concern of family members is for the safety of the patient, of the passengers in the patient's car, and, indeed, community members at large. Often, the concern extends beyond this to questions of liability and insurance coverage. I almost always feel that I am about to enter a family battle when at the end of the office visit I ask a senior patient if there are any questions and the son or daughter says, "Go ahead, Dad, ask him. Ask him if you can drive." The senior citizen then sheepishly asks about getting behind the wheel again, and everyone stares at me for the final word on whether the patient can safely drive. The truth of the matter is that I really don't know most of the time. I base my opinion on whether the person has been stable, whether laboratory tests show no major fluctuations, and whether there seems to be no susceptibility for sudden cardiac death. However, I think the issue is by and large one of liability, and I am usually reluctant to pronounce a level of safety for anyone to drive. I think this question should be resolved within the family after getting an opinion from the cardiologist or family doctor, but the final opinion does not, and should not, rest with the doctors.

Also, at the office visit, you should mention any medication you seem to be running low on and may run out of before the next office visit. In fact, you should ask when that office visit might be, and if the interval seems either too short or too long, you should inquire as to the reasoning. Use this visit to begin to get comfortable with your doctor, particularly if he or she is new to you. You might want to ask such specific questions as the following: When is a good time for me to make a phone call to your office? What is the best way to get a prescription refilled? What should I do if there is an emergency? Should I go to the closest hospital, or should I try to get to the hospital where you are on staff?

Many of my colleagues bristle at the idea of being called by their first name. I think at some point you ought to determine your doctor's preference about this—as well as reveal to him or her your preference on how you would like to be addressed. Remember that this is probably going to be a long-standing relationship between you and your doctor. Personally, I try to gauge what form of address my patients are comfortable with, and often I ask them. I think that doctors and nurses far too often assume a first-name intimacy and that this makes many patients, particularly the elderly, uncomfortable. On the other hand, using first names provides a sense of comfort for many patients and breaks down barriers. It's simply a matter of exercising good communication skills for doctors to inquire about this or to get a sense of it early on in a relationship. Patients have a similar responsibility. I have patients who call me by my first name; in fact, I think many of them do it as a sort of a test, to see what my reaction will be. Sometimes I detect other reasons. For example, a patient I saw two or three times, a gentleman who really had not been making much progress with his heart failure, suddenly addressed me by my first name. I immediately sensed that this was not an attempt to try to develop more of a friendship but an expression of his frustration with his lack of progress. I stopped the routine inquiries regarding his heart failure, looked at him, and asked, "What really seems to be bothering you the most?" He broke down and told me that he was concerned that he was probably going to die soon, since there was currently nothing that I could do for him. I told him that I had been trying to manage him quite conservatively because of his many associated medical conditions. It was at that point that he opened up and said, "Doc, I don't care what you have to do, but I've got to feel better than I do now or life is not worth living." We subsequently tried a more aggressive approach in his treatment, and, fortunately, it worked. Soon thereafter, I noticed that he was addressing me as Dr. Silver again. I mentioned this to him, he apologized for having called me by my first name, we had a long talk about our preferences, and I believe we arrived at an agreement with which both of us feel comfortable. The point is, the "correct" names for the doctor and the patient are the ones with which they are comfortable. As always, nothing compares with good communication and discussion.

As you can see, there are many issues that need to be addressed during each office visit. In the treatment of heart failure patients, a visit often results in changes in therapy or a reevaluation of the treatment strategy, which elicit a new and longer list of questions from the patient at the following visit. Perhaps that is why I enjoy treating patients with heart failure so much. There is really very little status quo. Patients do not stay stable for months or years at a time; they are either getting better or getting worse. I enjoy the challenge of getting everyone to make progress and move forward.

I think you can use the suggestions made in this chapter to take control over some aspect of your heart failure, to gain a better understanding of your treatments and your doctor's plans for you, and to help ensure that you stay out of the hospital and make the best use of your outpatient visits.

15

The Young Person
with Heart Failure

I recently heard a shocking statistic: Every seven seconds a baby-boomer turns fifty! As I approach that age group with rapid-fire speed, I am aware that my definition of a "young person" is evolving. Nevertheless, I am reminded daily that I am increasingly seeing new patients and taking care of those who are younger than what we normally consider the elderly of our nation.

The majority of patients in this country who have heart failure are over the age of sixty-five. That is not to say, however, that the younger patient is immune to serious heart disease or heart failure. The comments in this book apply to heart failure patients of any age. There are, however, special forms of heart failure that the younger patient may have:

1. Cardiomyopathy due to congenital heart disease
2. Alcohol-induced cardiomyopathy
3. Dilated cardiomyopathy with or without myocarditis
4. Diabetic cardiomyopathy
5. Familial cardiomyopathy
6. Chemotherapy-related cardiomyopathy
7. Cardiomyopathy due to premature coronary artery disease (heart attacks) or severe hypertension
8. AIDS-related cardiomyopathy
9. Peripartum cardiomyopathy

Obviously, with the exception of peripartum cardiomyopathy, these are forms of heart failure that can develop in people at any age, but some of these distinct forms tend to occur in younger patients. For example, although diabetic cardiomyopathy can certainly occur in any individual who has diabetes, studies have shown that diabetics on insulin, compared to nondiabetics, have a 2.4-fold higher incidence of developing heart failure and that this generally occurs at a younger age. Similarly, alcohol-related cardiomyopathy can occur at any age, but a patient with new onset of heart failure who has an alcohol abuse pattern related to it is frequently in his or her twenties, thirties, or forties.

In a moment I will discuss some of the specific forms, but there are some interesting statistics surrounding the younger patient with heart failure. It has long been known that older age gives a worse prognosis for patients with heart failure, but I am not convinced that younger age generally connotes a better prognosis. For example, according to one of the large heart failure databases (Studies on Left Ventricular Dysfunction [SOLVD] Registry), patients older than the age of seventy-six have a greater than 38 percent one-year mortality rate. Patients from ages twenty-one to fifty-five, however, have only a 16.6 percent mortality rate for the same one-year period. These statistics reflect a shorter period or duration of heart failure in younger individuals, or less serious disease. Since many younger individuals tend to get forms of heart failure that are reversible, the statistics reflect the greater likelihood of spontaneous remission or attenuation in these patients. For example, a young person with an undiagnosed case of myocarditis may have rather severe heart failure within the first year, but the condition may progressively improve or stabilize, and a large percentage of young women with peripartum cardiomyopathy, which I will discuss shortly, return completely to normal function. Moreover, although I mentioned earlier that there is a major increase in death from heart failure in this country, one of the few groups in which there has been a decline is white patients under the age of forty-five. The exact reasons for this decline and for the racial differences in susceptibility of this age group are unclear at the present time.

When I see young persons with severe heart failure, I always think of the many productive years they should have ahead of them and I redouble my efforts to find a reversible cause for their heart failure and to seek therapies that will not only make a major functional improvement in their lifestyle and quality of life but also prolong their lives.

COMMON PATHWAYS TO HEART FAILURE IN THE YOUNG

Young patients who have heart failure develop it from one of four common pathways. A young patient may have congenital heart disease, or a heart defect from birth; both individuals whose heart defect was surgically repaired and those whose defect was never detected may have heart damage, with long-term malfunction of the heart muscle leading to heart failure.

Another common situation is the development of a form of dilated cardiomyopathy (weak heart muscle). For example, young people may have bouts of myocarditis, or inflammation of the heart muscle, which may ultimately lead to a dilated cardiomyopathy. Or they may develop a spontaneous case of dilated cardiomyopathy, which we see all too frequently. According to some studies, up to 80 percent of all new cases of heart failure in young patients are due to idiopathic dilated cardiomyopathy, which means that the exact cause is unknown. A dilated cardiomyopathy in young patients is often directly related to alcohol abuse. Alcohol is a direct toxin (or damaging substance) to the heart muscle. Excessive alcohol can cause a severe weakness of the heart, but, with early cessation, the heart muscle function often returns to normal. As the abuse continues for longer periods of time, however, the damage becomes irreversible. I often see young men and women who drink more than a case of beer each weekend and then wonder why they have developed heart disease. This is an important, and potentially preventable, form of heart failure.

There is also a rare form of dilated cardiomyopathy that seems to be familial (that is, it runs in families) and frequently affects young patients. Often in these familial cases there is some specific defect, such as an abnormality in the mitochondria (tiny powerplants in all our cells that create the energy necessary to perform work) or a genetic deficiency in a substance such as carnitine (a substance the body uses to help burn fatty acids or fats as fuel for the muscles).

Unfortunately, despite educational efforts regarding the need to control blood pressure, stop smoking, and reduce cholesterol in the diet, we still see many young people who have advanced forms of coronary artery disease and even develop heart attacks. In the past, when I saw a forty-year-old with new heart failure, I would rarely consider doing an angiogram to see if the patient had coronary artery disease, but in the last five or six years, I've encountered severe coronary disease in young patients in their twenties and thirties often enough that I now frequently consider the possibility of a heart attack even in this age group. Although some of these patients have familiar forms of high levels of cholesterol and have specific forms of coronary artery disease, others have simply engaged in self-abusive behavior like smoking cigarettes and maintaining a high-fat diet, starting at a young age. So the young person who has suffered one or more heart attacks is certainly susceptible to developing heart failure.

Finally, one of the more unfortunate forms of heart failure that develop in a young person is what we call peripartum cardiomyopathy. Some young women, either during their last three months of pregnancy or within the first three months after delivery, are susceptible to developing what we call peripartum cardiomyopathy, the exact cause of which has not yet been determined. Because the disease tends to appear in somewhat less affluent populations, nutritional deficiency has been suggested as the cause. Other suggested causes include toxemia, very high blood pressure developing during pregnancy, antibodies (the immune system of the body attacking itself), an allergic reaction to certain drugs, and genetic susceptibility. Black women have a higher incidence of peripartum cardiomyopathy than white women, and advanced maternal age, numerous past pregnancies, and twin pregnancies seem to predispose women to this disease. However, I would like to emphasize that there really is no way to predict who might develop this disease; in my own experience, I have seen a preponderance of women who are white, pregnant for the first time, with a single baby, and with none of the other predisposing factors just mentioned. Inflammation of the heart muscle, or myocarditis, is commonly suspected as the cause of this form of cardiomyopathy. In one study, fourteen of eighteen women who had this cardiomyopathy were shown to have myocarditis on a biopsy of the heart muscle. Often, however, we find no cause whatsoever. The bad news is that this can be a serious form of cardiomyopathy; in fact, it can be fatal. On the other hand, many women do recover.

From various studies and my own personal experience, I would say that there is complete recovery in one-third of women with this disease, with one-third stabilizing and one-third dying from it. In the latter, there is often overwhelming myocarditis. Although we frequently try to discourage subsequent pregnancies in women who have had this disease, with very careful testing we can determine which women can deliver babies in the future without any difficulty. We do know that a woman who has had a peripartum cardiomyopathy is at high risk for worsening heart failure with subsequent pregnancies. However, because of their young age, many of these women do want to consider additional pregnancies. In that case, I usually recommend a minimum period of two years from the time of the cardiomyopathy to allow for an adequate period of stabilization and observation. During that time, I watch the patient carefully to make sure she has no early symptomatic recurrence of her heart failure. If she is completely stable and asymptomatic over that period of time, I make several measurements, including either an echocardiogram or MUGA, to follow the overall function of the left ventricle. I also commonly rely on CPX testing to determine how the heart muscle may respond during pregnancy, which places a variety of stresses on even a normal heart. Since it is important to gauge how the extra blood volume and energy requirements of a pregnancy may affect a previously damaged heart muscle, the overall efficiency and ability to exercise adequately on the CPX test is one of the measurements I rely on before condoning a young woman's decision to become pregnant again after she has suffered peripartum cardiomyopathy.

CHEMOTHERAPY-RELATED CARDIOMYOPATHY

Certain forms of chemotherapy, or drugs used to fight cancers, can cause serious heart muscle damage and heart failure. The risk for developing heart muscle damage seems to be related to the total dose of medication received (usually adriamycin), the combination of other heart-damaging chemotherapeutic agents, such as high doses of cyclophosphamide, and radiation treatment for the tumor. This type of cardiomyopathy is commonly seen today in younger women who have undergone chemotherapy for breast cancer, but it is also commonly seen in patients who received these treatments for various forms of lymphoma. It is a very sad situation when a young patient who has licked one serious disease develops another because of the treatment received. Often this form of heart failure develops suddenly; unfortunately, it is usually a progressive and eventually fatal form of heart failure. Cancer specialists and cardiologists are working closer together nowadays to better study the heart muscle after each round of chemotherapy in hopes of preventing heart failure due to the cancer treatment and to develop alternative therapies that can be given to people who are susceptible to this kind of damage. If you are getting chemotherapy with adriamycin, you may want to keep track of the total dose you have received, because the overall risk of damage to the heart muscle increases greatly beyond a certain threshold. If you have had any prior cardiac history, including high blood pressure or prior heart attack, you may be more susceptible to the development of heart failure while undergoing treatment with anticancer drugs.

AIDS AND HEART FAILURE

Finally, there is a great deal of media attention on the epidemic of AIDS, which continues to take approximately 50,000 lives annually in the United States. I am frequently asked about the relationship between AIDS, heart disease, and heart failure. AIDS tends predominantly to affect young people, and some of the early research I did at the National Institutes of Health was on the cardiac involvement in young patients who died of AIDS. What we found initially was that Kaposi's sarcoma, a blood vessel tumor, occurs in patients with AIDS and affects the heart. Shortly thereafter, we found that there is also inflammation of the heart muscle, or a form of myocarditis, in these young patients. Today, it is widely recognized that the heart is commonly involved in patients who have AIDS, and as often as 50 percent of the time, myocarditis is found in the heart of an AIDS victim. Heart involvement can present in a variety of ways, including inflammation of the lining of the heart, fluid between the two layers of the heart, inflammation of the heart muscle, and even infection of the heart valves. Suffice it to say that heart failure is not uncommon in patients with AIDS and usually coexists with other forms of disability. Overall, it has been estimated that between 2 and 10 percent of patients with AIDS will develop congestive heart failure related to their illness. There has not been any evidence that links the development of heart failure with how a patient contracted AIDS, but one study suggests that patients with lower counts of certain white blood cells, or infection-fighting cells, are most susceptible.

There are particular treatment dilemmas in treating patients with AIDS. One of the ways we try to treat inflammation in the heart muscle of patients in general is by suppressing the person's immune system. The patient with AIDS already has a suppressed immune system, and ongoing studies are trying to determine if further immunosuppression is beneficial or detrimental. Also, some of the drug therapies used to treat AIDS patients may in fact cause a form of heart failure. It is this effect of the drug AZT that may limit its use in patients with AIDS.

SPECIAL CONSIDERATIONS WITH THE YOUNGER PATIENT

Regardless of the cause of heart failure in young patients, basically the same approach is applied to them in terms of trying to discover the cause, estimate the prognosis, initiating the proper drug therapy, and then fine-tuning the dosage. However, there are some special considerations in the case of the young person who has heart failure, in contrast to the seventy-five-year-old. Probably one of the most obvious differences is that not only are we trying to achieve the goals mentioned in previous chapters regarding improved survival, functional improvement, and a better quality of life, but we are also interested in sustaining all of these benefits over an extended period of time.

It is especially painful to see a young person with advanced heart failure, because we know that we may not be able to help him or her live into maturity. It is sometimes more difficult for me to approach young patients who have heart failure. Frequently, they must go from a stage in which they must accept the fact that they are temporarily sick and may be off work for a while to a stage in which they must face the fact that they have a life-threatening disease and that it is not only their years of livelihood that might be cut short, but also their life span. I go out of my way to provide hope and help for these young patients in particular, but I can honestly say that the loss of a young patient to heart failure is certainly one of the most painful experiences I go through. I think that this potential for premature death is one of the strongest motives in referring a patient to a transplant program rather quickly. As we have discussed earlier, however, the long waiting times for transplantation and the lack of donors limit transplantation as an option. Also, we need to recall that transplantation may not be truly a permanent solution. It won't allow a twenty-year-old to reach the ripe old age of seventy or eighty, but may allow them to live to forty. Also, it involves many quality-of-life issues, especially for a younger patient. Fortunately, we are getting better at determining who might need a transplant; we now base our decisions on information provided by such testing as the CPX test rather than rely only on functional status or ejection fractions.

Another thing to consider for the young patient is the lifestyle that person leads. The eighty-year-old, seventy-year-old, or even sixty-year-old may be able to retire or certainly will not have a daily requirement to get up and go to work. Retirement may not be possible for the younger patient with heart failure, which presents an additional worry and burden to the patient and family members. Frequently, the spouse has to find a job to maintain the family's lifestyle, and I've seen several young families undergo major changes because of this. The steps required to get financial assistance usually require using up all other family assets, and this only serves to further demoralize and break apart the family unit. The young person with heart failure certainly requires as much emotional and psychological support as the elderly patient, perhaps even more, since the latter has had some time to adjust to a more limited lifestyle. It is also difficult to explain to children why their mother or father cannot be as active with them as they were before.

Because of the suddenness with which heart failure comes on in some young patients, there is frequently a period of disbelief, anger, and often even refusal to accept all the treatments that are necessary. With alcohol- or cocaine-related cardiomyopathy, this reaction may be related to the substance abuse itself, but usually it is a reflection of the young person's sense of immortality. Great anguish accompanies the clash between this youthful sense of immortality and the harsh reality of personal mortality that must be faced by the young person with any serious disease, including heart failure. Fortunately, there are support groups, such as Young Hearts, an organization founded in the Chicago area (see Appendix II), so that younger patients can discuss common issues with a group of peers. Since the issues facing younger and older patients differ, it is important to have support groups that focus on one or the other age group, so that group members receive the specific emotional support and counseling needed for their form of heart disease.

CONCLUSION

Young persons with heart failure truly represent a special situation. They are special in terms of the forms of heart failure they get as well as the socioeconomic problems that go with their heart failure. The aims and goals for treatment of these patients are also different. I must emphasize the importance of support and education for younger patients with heart failure. They may be at a stage in life when they have not yet started a family and may lack strong social support. They are often overwhelmed by fears of being sick and thoughts of mortality. I feel strongly that every effort should be made to find a reversible cause for heart failure in every patient, but this is especially so in the case of the younger patient. We must guide these patients to a better understanding of their disease so that they can seek treatment, accept help, and learn to lead active, productive lives despite often significant physical limitations. I believe that treating the younger patient with heart failure is one of the great challenges we must face.

16

For Families Only

I remember one particular occasion when I first saw a new patient who was eighty years old. She came to the office accompanied by two loving daughters and a son. We spent a great deal of time discussing her heart failure and the other treatments she had received. I told her quite honestly that there were many things we could try and that I felt there was great hope for some improvement in how she felt and in her ability to do more. You could see the light come on in this woman's face. I looked at her children, who were all nodding their heads in agreement and presenting courteous smiles on their faces, but when I got up to leave the room, they followed me out into the hallway. One of them said, "Doc, thanks so much for giving her that encouragement. It's nice to see her smile again," but then said, "Now, Doc, tell us what's really going to happen to Mom." I told them the same thing I tell every family member who follows me out into the hall or who calls me back the following day: I do not say anything to patients that I do not think is true. I honestly believe there is hope and help for almost everyone with heart failure.

Yes, there are patients for whom I feel nothing more can be done. I usually tell them so quite honestly, although they often suspect it long before I tell them. I do not believe in either overinflating or hiding from a patient any of the realities of his or her prognosis. After all, these individuals are my patients, and it is to them that I must communicate the good and the bad, but always the truth. The point is that most doctors are quite honest with their patients, and unless you suspect that a doctor is saying some things to your family member for moral support alone, I do not recommend that you follow the doctor out into the hall or corner him or her outside the hospital room and whisper about your family member. This only puts doubt in the mind of the patient. When family members approach me in this way, I frequently take them back into the room in front of the patient, readdress their concerns, and state once again that I do not say anything to the family that I wouldn't say directly to the patient. I think that family members can be very supportive of their sick relative by asking their questions and stating their concerns in the presence of the patient.

I think there are many other ways that families can be supportive of and extremely helpful to the patient with heart failure. These are ways in addition to helping patients shop, get their medications, visit the library to obtain more information about their heart problem, or write to the American Heart Association. One of the things I frequently tell my patients and their families is to discuss among themselves what they want done in the event of an emergency, that is, if the person has a cardiac arrest. Does the patient want to be resuscitated? Does he or she want to be on a ventilator? I also encourage patients and their families to discuss the concept of a living will. They usually don't make all of these decisions by themselves—I think that for many families and patients, this is a pretty difficult experience—but at least this topic gets them going on the road to communicating with one another once again. I think it also serves to emphasize that heart failure is a serious disease. Many families need to be made aware of this and need to learn to talk to one another again in loving and caring ways. Knowing that the ill family member may not be around within the next year or so can sometimes break down the anger that has unknowingly built up over the years. Trivial events in the past can now be overshadowed by current needs, if families just let them. Families must bear the responsibility of being the patient's major source of support. It is not the responsibility of hospitals, other institutions, or doctors. The major source of support for the patient must come from the family.

One concept that Dr. Bernie Siegel makes perfectly clear in his writings is that people—patients and families—need to understand that death comes to everyone. And that death is not a failure. It is not a failure of the person who suffers with the disease, it is not a failure of the family, it is not a failure of the doctor, and it is not a failure of modern medicine. It is simply the inevitable failure of the body, and when everything has been done that can be done, people need to face death not as a failure of their ability to live but with rejoicing for the life they have had. Nor do I view as failures those patients who have severe heart failure because they ate too much fat and cholesterol, smoked too many cigarettes, or drank too much in their younger years. If they can control these habits now and take control over their disease by learning about their medications and educating themselves about fluid and salt restriction, then they are in fact successes. Who among us has done everything right all the time? We all make mistakes, and more than anything else, our ability to communicate, to touch souls with one another, is what makes us successful. Family members are in a position to make the greatest contribution to this communication.

Although communicating early with a patient should be a two-way street, all too often it starts out as a one-way affair. Worse than that, nobody knows whose job it is to start the flow of communication. It would be wonderful if all patients who had heart failure could reach out and talk to their family and tell them what they were going through, but this is often very difficult to do. The reason I hear most often from my patients is that they don't want to burden their spouse, their son, their daughter, their grandchildren. Therefore, the patient frequently remains silent. On the other hand, family members themselves are often reluctant to start communicating because they think the patient is weak, tired, or just not up to a long-winded conversation. Most important, many people suffer anxiety when faced with the need to confront the subject of death.

I remember treating a middle-aged woman who had been very active until she developed a serious form of heart failure. When she first came to see me, her two children were eighteen and twenty, and she still enjoyed picking out special Christmas presents for them. As her heart failure got worse and her energy level dropped, she found that she had less and less energy for her special shopping at Christmastime each year. At first, she would pick out whatever she could find in a single store, and later she found herself just giving money to the children as presents. I could tell from her comments to me that she felt great pain in no longer being able to buy presents for her children. Furthermore, she was not able to have an open conversation with them and say, "Look, kids, I really am being affected by my illness. I love you just as much but simply can't get out to buy the presents any more. Do you understand?" On the other hand, her children, who probably didn't care what she got them for presents, were also unable to open up the conversation and say, "Look, Mom, we know that you are tired more and have less energy. It is not the Christmas presents that we're concerned about; we're just happy that you're here with us. What can we do to make life easier for you?"

Now, every family's dynamics are different, but husbands and wives, fathers and sons, and mothers and daughters all have special relationships to one another. I don't think that doctors or nurses—or even psychologists or psychiatrists—can have the impact on patients that family members can have simply by communicating with them. That is why I've written this chapter. I'd like to see one party or the other—patient or family—start the one-way communication and pursue it until it becomes a two-way street where conversation, laughter, and tears are going back and forth across it.

I mentioned earlier that whether a heart failure patient continues to drive is a decision that needs to be made by patients and their family, and not really by the doctor. Yes, ask the doctor what he or she thinks about driving for the patient, but in the end, it is going to have to be a family decision. Another decision that frequently has to be made concerns the patient's living accommodations. Frequently, elderly patients who have heart failure (or any disease, for that matter) need to make a change in their environment. Perhaps they need to find an apartment that is on the first floor because they cannot walk up the stairs any longer, or they need to move in with a son or daughter because they can't manage on their own. These kinds of decisions are tough at best but are almost always reached more easily when families can sit down together and discuss the pros and cons; under such circumstances, a solution that is amenable to all is more likely to be hammered out. We do not need Henry Kissinger to come into our family kitchens and living rooms, but simply a willingness to understand what the family member with heart failure is going through, what his or her needs are, and what we as family members can do to help.

Probably one of the most important ways I have seen families support patients with heart failure is by helping them set goals and priorities. Probably one of the hardest passages there is for young men and women who watch an elderly parent grow old, get sick, and approach death is to change roles in the parent-child relationship and assume the role of caretaker. Having to address questions regarding nursing homes, home care, and even funeral arrangements are important steps that patients and families can take together. The family can help by setting positive goals. One of the most remarkable patients I care for is a ninety-three-year-old man whose wife is one of the most positive influences I have ever seen. She is fortunate to have her health, but instead of bemoaning how ill her husband is and how limited he is, she continues to plan excursions, jaunts, and goals for him. Every time they come into the office, she says something like, "Well, we just got back from our granddaughter's wedding in Iowa, and now we are planning to attend our grandson's birthday in Michigan." Every time they come in, she has a new goal for him. Continuing to establish short- and medium-term goals for patients with heart failure is, I think, one of the most important functions families can serve.

Finally, let me say that whether or not you think your family has strong emotional bonds, families are the basis of our emotional selves. So I urge families to get involved, to talk to their loved ones, to investigate what can be done for the member with heart failure, and to give that person a hug or simply express love and support for him or her. Family members not only need to help sick members make decisions regarding investigational trials and get their medicines but also take charge of their health through empowerment rather than to allow others to treat them like a dependent child.

It is interesting that some of the strongest family support comes to patients who are the sickest with their heart failure. Now, this probably does not surprise you, but I'll tell you why it surprises me. As I think about some of my sickest patients, I think that many of them are among the most fortunate. Despite their serious illness, they have tremendous support and understanding from their families. I am thinking of one woman in particular who has outlived virtually everyone's expectations for her, including my own. Now, this patient's family could simply coddle her and restrict her activities, and be well justified in doing so. However, they have learned from both the patient and me that she is going to have good days and bad days with her illness. She also has an openness and willingness to communicate to her family when she is having a good day and when she is having a bad one. Both patient and family take full advantage of the good days, and I frequently hear not only about the days when my patient is sick and requires additional medication but also about the days when she is out in the shopping mall, even if she has to be pushed in a wheelchair. The point is that she is in control and, along with her family, makes the decisions from day to day.

Other patients who are not nearly as limited may have families whose members simply concentrate on the heart failure. They prescribe their own brand of well-intentioned limitations that only serve to demoralize and decondition the patient even more. They have not made a full effort to understand the disease their loved one has, and as a result, they are doing them a disservice. I believe this approach is often adopted out of love for the sick member, but at the same time, it reveals a fear of ongoing communication.

I am reminded of the story of the young man named Lorenzo Odone. You may have seen the wonderful movie called *Lorenzo's Oil,* which portrays the endless fight Lorenzo's mother and father put up in their effort to find a treatment for the rare nervous system disease he had. These parents loved their child, but what parent does not? The difference here is that these parents showed affection for their son by getting to know everything they could about his disease and struggling with him to find a cure.

SUMMARY

In summary, family members can help a patient with heart failure enormously. They can help in obvious ways, such as picking up medications, giving the patient a ride, or simply helping with the grocery shopping. I think, however, the most important way family members can help is by making sure the patient who suffers with heart failure does not suffer alone. Get to know about the disease and what can be done for it, and become a true partner for your family member who suffers. It is with this kind of communication and love that the suffering comes to an end and the healing truly begins.

17

The Fearsome Twosome:
Pulmonary Hypertension and Sudden Death

There are a couple of areas in heart failure that don't seem to get discussed much; well, at least, not between patients and doctors. I have always felt this is because these areas are ones of great frustration and perhaps even misunderstanding for most physicians. I'd like to say a few words about these so that you can never say I didn't bring up the topic, you did hear about it in this book, and I can give you my perspectives.

PULMONARY HYPERTENSION

I will start with pulmonary hypertension. Basically, as I have explained before, this is simply high blood pressure in the blood vessels of the lungs. There are several different forms of pulmonary hypertension, but it is usually broken down into primary pulmonary hypertension and secondary pulmonary hypertension. In the first, there are abnormalities in the lung arteries without, as yet, a known cause. This disease affects all types of people but especially young people, with a slight preponderance of women. There are an estimated 2 million people so affected.

The other forms of pulmonary hypertension are the result of other diseases. One of the most common causes is congestive heart failure but they can also be seen in other cardiac diseases, such as mitral valve disease and some forms of congenital heart disease, and other noncardiac diseases such as collagen vascular diseases.

Regardless of the cause or type, this is indeed problematic, since progressively increasing pressures in the lungs create more pressure and work for the right side of the heart, which is not built to withstand such high pressures. When the right ventricle fails, there is a marked limitation in exercise, with fluid accumulation in the gut and in the legs.

The reason pulmonary hypertension is not talked about is that often it is thought to be difficult, if not impossible, to treat and its presence usually signals the end stages of disease. I have always been aggressive in both measuring and treating pulmonary hypertension, and so I seem to have less fear of its presence. One of the ways to measure the degree of pulmonary hypertension is to place a right heart catheter, or Swan-Ganz catheter, which allows direct measurement of the pressure. Once in place, a variety of medications can be tried that may alter the blood pressure inside the lungs. Recently, a newer form of medication called prostacylin or Flolan has become available and is often effective for treatment. In fact, although this is an intravenous drug, patients with primary pulmonary hypertension have been shown to have significant improvement and lessened mortality when getting this drug through a constant infusion. For some reason, when infusion of the same drug was tried with heart failure patients, there seemed to be an increase of mortality. Fortunately, many other drugs work for heart failure patients, and usually I can find some way to improve patients' pulmonary hypertension and relieve their symptoms of right heart failure.

Clearly, all the issues surrounding pulmonary hypertension are not yet known. However, I strongly believe that often something can be done to improve or reverse the pulmonary hypertension and should always be tried. This is one area that I feel you need an aggressive medical team to address. Ultimately, with the development of newer, orally active agents, this problem should be considered right along with the others of the failing heart.

There is a wonderful support group, originally only for patients with the primary form of pulmonary hypertension. Lately, they are working to educate and raise awareness for the secondary forms of the disease as well. I suggest you contact them for more information and join as a member; they have a great newsletter *(Pathlight)*. Send them a contribution—it's worth it.

Pulmonary Hypertension Association
P.O. Box 24733
Speedway, Indiana 46224-0733
Phone: (800) 748-7274
Internet: www.phassociation.com

SUDDEN DEATH

Wow, talk about a bad name—and you thought heart failure was a bad choice. All kidding aside, this is a serious problem, since sudden death is the mode of death in approximately 30 to 50 percent of patients with heart failure. Usually, this is due to the sudden onset of an irregular, fast heartbeat called ventricular tachycardia or ventricular fibrillation. About 30 percent of the time, however, sudden death is proven to be due to a slow or absent heartbeat (bradyarrhythmia). The weakened and scarred heart is a perfect setup for these irregularities in the heartbeat. Interestingly, the worse the ejection fraction and, in my experience, the worse the level of decompensation, such as fluid accumulation, the greater the risk of sudden death.

Now you might think from the term *sudden death* that a person has only a single episode of this and does not survive. Fortunately, some episodes do terminate and the patient survives after having an episode of syncope, or passing out. Often, they are cardioverted or shocked in the field by paramedics, or even make it to the emergency room. Sometimes people have ventricular tachycardia and yet do not pass out and even walk themselves into the hospital. Those people I just mentioned are the lucky ones, those cases that can be detected and survive their episode of sudden cardiac death. Also, for them, it is quite clear that they are likely to have other episodes and may benefit from having a defibrillator inserted.

A defibrillator, now placed easily as a pacemaker and connected via a lead or electrode without major surgery, can detect irregular heartbeat and respond in a variety of ways, including trying to pace the heart out of an irregular heartbeat before applying an internal shock. It is clear that these are remarkable and life-saving devices, and in certain groups, they need to be used more widely.

The problem of sudden death, however, is that we are not sure most of the time who is likely to develop sudden death, and even less is known about what is exactly the right treatment. We know that certain antiarrhythmia drugs can actually worsen the risk of sudden death, whereas others may be useful in its prevention.

Just to show you the lack of knowledge we have regarding treatment, a good friend of mine, Dr. Gust Bardy, has designed a large national trial called SCDHeFT (Sudden Cardiac Death in Heart Failure Trial) precisely to look at this issue. In this trial, patients who had symptomatic heart failure and are already on good heart failure medicine are getting randomized into one of three groups (no medication or device, a medicine called amiodarone, or the installation of a defibrillator device). I hope this study will answer the question regarding the best way to prevent heart failure deaths due to sudden death. By the way, patients with pulmonary hypertension often experience sudden deaths as well.

Personally, when I lose a patient to sudden death, I feel so hopeless in having been unable to prevent it. Also, I readily admit that I often did not speak to patients about the possibility of sudden death. It was not until the pilot study we performed to get ready for the SCDHeFT trial that I got more into the habit of discussing this major problem. I still just wish we had a better name!

I think that you should be aware of the sudden death issue in heart failure, and don't be afraid to address it with your doctors and nurses. Often, getting it out into the open for discussion takes away some of the fear.

Although we have more information about the value of defibrillators in patients who have had a heart attack, the use of defibrillators in all patients with heart failure (prophylaxis) remains a cloudy issue. Stay tuned for better news in the future about both of these problems. Tremendous minds and research dollars are focusing on these serious problems with the failing heart.

18

The Future of Heart Failure

This is always the hardest chapter to write. In all the other chapters, I am able to write about what is and what has been. Now, this is my turn to try and predict the future—something I'm rarely great at, try as I might! When I talk with my patients about some of the prognostic indicators with heart failure, I remind them that I do not have a crystal ball and cannot see what lies down the road for them. I tell them that we use the prognostic indicators as a guide to where they might be in the near future. I think looking at the future possibilities and probabilities for heart failure treatment is much the same. And if you asked 100 health professionals in this country about how heart failure will be treated in the next decade, you might well get 100 different answers. However, in this chapter I'd like to highlight what I think are some of the future trends in approaching heart failure, at least over the next decade or so.

First and foremost, I think the medical approach to heart failure is going to be driven by a socioeconomic force sooner rather than later. Because of the ever-increasing number of patients with heart failure and the enormous economic burden to our health care system, as well as to the finances of individual families, heart failure is gaining a lot of attention at both national and local political levels. To some extent, this philosophy has already occurred. Since I wrote the first edition, there are now three different textbooks of heart failure, three new heart failure journals, and even our own Heart Failure Society.

I believe heart failure will be one of the disease processes that will be targeted to require that physicians demonstrate that some of the treatments we currently use actually impact outcomes. As applied to heart failure, *outcome* is a word with political and socioeconomic connotations that include not only all of the goals I mentioned before, including longevity, functional ability, and quality of life, but also the idea of the economic cost of caring for patients with heart failure. I think we should welcome this outcome-based approach as long as the initial goals are emphasized and everything is not reduced to a simple bottom line.

For many years, I have told other doctors that it is my opinion that heart failure is an outpatient disease. Considering that the number one cause for hospitalization of patients over the age of sixty-five is heart failure, they find my statement hard to believe. However, as we move closer to adopting an outcome-driven approach to heart failure, we will increasingly find that more and more patients can be managed in an outpatient setting and that the number of hospital admissions for these patients will be markedly reduced. How this can happen is suggested in many of the chapters in this book.

In terms of diagnosis of heart failure, I think we will continue to emphasize the importance of finding the etiology accurately, since there will probably be better specific treatments for heart failure based on particular etiologies. I am certain that we will have better high-tech ways of sorting out the nonspecific diagnosis of dilated cardiomyopathy into more specific diagnoses that can be accurately assessed and treated. I think we will find better ways to diagnose myocarditis as well as familial forms of dilated cardiomyopathy, and in the not too distant future, we'll probably use gene therapy to treat and even prevent some of the hereditary forms of heart failure. I also think that we are going to be able to identify some of the early forms of heart failure with noninvasive methods and therefore start treatments for patients when they are not quite so sick, thus allowing us to make a major impact on the long-term morbidity and mortality of patients.

In terms of medical treatments, advances will come in several forms. We will continue to learn more about how heart failure develops from an early asymptomatic stage to a stage of overt symptomatology. We will attack the disease with a multidimensional method using what Dr. Jay Cohn has called *polypharmacy.* I believe that in only a few short years, we'll probably be using as standard therapy four and maybe five drugs to treat heart failure (and we can only wonder what impact that will have on the economic burden of treating our patients). I believe that there will be many advances in the field of transplantation, primarily coming with the development of a totally implantable artificial heart, which will avoid the current problems of donor shortage and requirements for immunosuppression. There will also be some advances made in the area of *xenotransplantation,* that is, using animals to supply a heart for a needy human. Actually, scientists are already well along with a swine (pig) model that should be able to provide organs for human transplantation without causing severe immune rejection problems.

We will also see increased interest in nonpharmacological methods of treating heart failure. There will be greater attention at all levels of medical care to some of the basics, such as fluid and salt restriction, and many programs will develop to encourage exercise training as a form of therapy for patients with heart failure.

Currently, it is estimated that one-third of Americans have used alternative medical sources within this country at some time within the past year. I trust that our knowledge and investigation of alternative methods for treating heart failure will accelerate to provide some scientific support and guidance for what could otherwise become mass mania among our needy population. We will rediscover ancient and nutritional forms of treatment by doing our *re*-search properly. However, it is frightening to see government cuts for research spending at a time when we need good clinical and basic research more than ever.

I see in the very near future the wider application of long-term use of left ventricular assist devices both as destination and as bridge to recovery and these devices will continue to improve, reduce in size, be freer of infectious complications, and cost less!

We will continue to understand better the neurohormonal soup the failing heart is bathed in and develop drugs that better block and turn off these bad humors and thereby slow down disease progression. Then, with gene therapy, we will be able to rebuild damaged heart muscle—something never thought possible to do. Also, on a molecular level, we will understand better the process of hypertrophy and growth, and find better ways to modulate it and turn off excessive and unfavorable growth.

Going out on a limb, I believe we will merge along research lines with the cancer researchers to discover that the ultimate avenue of preventing and treating heart failure is by control of the normal and abnormal vasculature or blood vessels. All the action in the heart is ultimately seen in the heart muscle and its connecting collagen network, but the silent gatekeepers, I believe, are the tiny, quiet, but hardworking blood vessels that are really dealt the initial blows and injuries and respond with a variety of responses that initiate and ultimately lead to the syndrome that we call heart failure.

Finally a word about prevention, which I believe is the ultimate way to treat heart failure, that is, to prevent it from ever occurring. At a recent lecture I gave at a geriatric cardiology symposium, I ended the lecture with two slides that read: THE CURE FOR HEART FAILURE IN THE ELDERLY . . . IS PREVENTION OF CARDIOVASCULAR DISEASE IN THE YOUNG. In fact, the only cure we will ever have for heart failure lies in preventing the multiple forms of heart and lung disease that precede its development. We certainly are making advances in this country in terms of lowering the incidence of heart attack and stroke, but the problems still loom large. We must not forget that cardiovascular disease still kills more Americans than any other disease. We must totally rethink how we live and work in order to find ways to prevent cardiovascular disease, which attacks even our very young.

These are goals that will take decades to have an impact, but we must start now. We must convince industry and government that we care about our health and that of our loved ones. We must start now to wage a war on unhealthy behavior in general; only then will we have an impact on the health of this nation and finally have success with heart failure.

19

CHF@Internet.com

AUTHOR'S NOTE

As I said in the last edition, I expected it to truly be the final edition I would write since I expected the Internet to provide so much more information to people. In many ways, the information has been made available but people, particularly older patients with heart failure, have not learned or do not have access to an Internet-connected computer.

However, I think that over the next few years this will change. Speaking of change, the Heart Failure web sites change so much that I cannot keep up with them, so I have left this chapter pretty much unchanged. I suggest you go to a web search engine (I love google.com) and type in heart failure . . . you will be on the path. Just remember that the information comes to you unfiltered so be sure to discuss what you find and learn with your doctors and nurses.

—MAS

You are holding the last version of this book I will write! Let me tell you why I believe this is so. As I mentioned in the introduction to this edition, my primary goal in writing a book about heart failure was to give my own patients and their families a guidebook about their disease. On a broader scale, I did hope to heighten public awareness about the heart failure epidemic and serve as a resource for information about this disease.

I believe that there is an ongoing information revolution—the amount of information available is doubling at a blazing speed, but even more important, how we get our information has changed. For example, I rarely read a newspaper for news, sports scores, or even weather reports. Rather, I can get the most current information whenever I need it by getting "on-line" with my computer. My children don't go to the library to do reports or even turn to a twenty-four-volume set of the *World Book Encyclopedia*. Rather, they get the information they need through the computer. Today, we can read a book, shop, chat, and even order our groceries and dinner electronically.

Now, I'll admit that I have been fascinated by computer technology from the outset, but by no means am I an expert, nor do I possess any special skills. But I think that more and more of us have access to a computer either at home, at work, or at a public site such as a library. With such access, coupled with the enormous increase in the amount of information, we derive heightened awareness of so many issues. I believe that one of the major impacts computerization has had, and will continue to have on us, is how we get and process health-related information.

Therefore, when I say that another edition of this book won't be needed, I say it because I think that over the next several years more and more patients will obtain the information differently; yes, still from doctors, nurses, hospitals, and so on, but it will be more focused information—attempts to focus on a topic they read about on the net.

Currently, I would guess that roughly 30 to 40 percent of my own patients use a computer either at work or at home, and most will use the Internet or e-mail. I always give a new patient my business card, which has my office e-mail address, and I'm less and less surprised when I get a question or report on their weight in my in-box the next morning. In reality, this is a very efficient way to communicate, with lots of caveats that I won't go into now (that is, lack of two-way dialogue, ability to document a medical decision, and so on).

As you would imagine, most of my patients are elderly, and for that reason the majority have not been exposed to computers and frequently lack the resources to get into the computer scene. However, I must tell you that some of the best electronic tracking of weights and medicines has been done by some seniors who have a computer spreadsheet, interest, and time to spare!

What probably will change the usage of computers in health care and health education over the next several years will be the following:

- I understand that a "baby-boomer" turns fifty every minute. What this means is that those who were exposed to computers in the home and workplace will have this familiarity of computer expertise when they begin to develop health problems.
- More exposure to computers in everyday life, such as in grocery stores, auto dealerships, restaurants, and so on, will decrease the level of intimidation toward their usage and acceptance.
- Web television, or the ability to get on-line with an electronic device that most are already comfortable with, will boom. If one can surf the net as easily as flip between television channels, then information flow will become a flood into millions of households worldwide.

The point of all this is that, over the next several years, it will be easy, cheap, and time efficient to get health-related information and services via computer. What about right now? Currently, one can find good information about many health conditions. Unfortunately, it is not always easy, and a lot of trial and error and hours of searching need to take place before one finds the information. Also, when you search the net, you need a pretty good filter in your brain to help you decipher what may be of value, what is questionable, and what is pure trash. As I've said before, when you get on the information highway, keep your eyes open and your pocketbooks closed!

Finally, there still needs to be a reasonable level of computer expertise or "geekiness" to get the information out. I trust that all this will change.

For now, however, in a very random, unorganized, and unstructured way, I'd like to share with you some of the web sites I have found that I believe can bring you more information about your health generally and heart failure specifically. Before I start, let me emphasize that I am not an expert, and this list is a very partial listing—really just sites I have found on my own. I cannot explain computers to you or tell you the difference between a URL and what HTML means, but there are books for that. Therefore, I assume you know how to turn on your computer, have an Internet service provider, and know a little about navigating the Internet. If not, find out and then come back and reexplore this chapter. Also, I do not guarantee the content of any site, its security, or that you'll even find it, but it sure is fun surfing the Heart Failure Net!

BEGINNING WEB SITES

One of the most common questions people write to me about is finding a heart failure expert in their locale. One of the best ways to get this information is to log on to the home page of your local university medical center or hospital. You'd be surprised by the number of persons who have their own "home page" these days. Since a home page or Internet site can provide so much information, and there really is no one policing what information goes onto the page, the Internet in most cases can be viewed as one large ad. For better or worse, when you access a site such as your local hospital, you may well find not only good health care information but also a Madison Avenue quality, with the hospital "puffing its wares" over the modem lines. Actually, this is okay with me in general, because if the hospital has a program or service it is proud of, then it is probably something you want to know about and at least check into further. Therefore, you may well find out that there is a local heart failure expert right in your own locale just by following a few keystrokes. The other warning, however, is that just because something is not mentioned doesn't mean it doesn't exist.

Often, the best programs just haven't had the time, money, or marketing skills to advertise electronically.

Perhaps the very best place to start is at the homepage of the Heart Failure Society of America (http://www.HFSA.org or www.abouthf.org). Here you'll find a ton of patient-related materials including several wonderful modules we are just creating on topics like salt, medications, exercise, and so forth. You will also be able to read the guidelines and decide if you are getting the best care. This site is truly terrific!

Another superb site for all kinds of general health information is Advocate Health Care, located at

http://www.advocatehealth.com

Some useful heart information is at

http://advocatehealth.com/sites/specialty/cht/index.html

Here, you will get an overview of the institution and the medical center, as well as information about doctors, locations, and so on. As I said, it's advertising. There are some general health topics to look up, but these frequently are canned little blurbs that are purchased as a service and generic in nature. Actually, there is some really good stuff within the Intranet (a private internal network), where you can access our own excellent CHF education materials, an on-line encyclopedia of drugs, and instructions for heart-related tests in English and Spanish. The secret code to get into the Intranet is . . . oops, sorry, can't do that, but sooner or later, this kind of information will be available more generally.

Sometimes you want some of the basics. For example, many patients who have had two or three bypass operations do not even know what was hooked up to what. Dr. Mark Levinson from Seattle helps run a terrific site called the Learning Center, and there you can access one of the best detailed explanations and color pictures of how coronary artery bypass surgery is done! Also at this site, you can really track some of the latest discussions regarding cardiac surgery. For example, papers on the Batista procedure can be read there. Start your visit at

http://www.hsforum.com/heartsurgery

The bypass article is located at

http://www.hsforum.com/heartsurgery/TLC/CABG/CABGTLC.hsf

A good, extensive health site is called Health World. Here, you can do free Medline searches, as well as find a heavy-duty approach to natural and alternative therapies for many diseases. Read it. You'll like it.

http://www.healthy.net

If you want to get started viewing several cardiology journals and their electronic presentations, then visit

http://www.pulsus.com/cardiol/links.htm

or

http://www.hrt.org/major.html

HEART FAILURE SITES

There are thousands of sites out there, some good, some not so good. Many are just advertising their program or products. But after an hour on the net, you will end up quite knowledgeable about heart failure.

I am not easily impressed by fancy web pages, but I am impressed by content. For about a year now, I have followed what I think is the big mama of all heart failure web pages, simply because it has such good content—current and fairly accurate. And it's all run by a gentleman named Jon, who has heart failure. He is a computer whiz and the site has great music, as well as pictures of his family and their pets, but again, it's got content, content, content. There are many links, as I'll explain. First, start at Jon's Place:

http://www.chfpatients.com or www.jonsplace.org

There's a glossary that's quite good and, as I said, links galore. Explore his Kitchen Corner and discover some basic as well as high-tech tips on low-sodium cooking. Also linked from this page—in fact, how I got here in the first place searching for CoEnzyme Q_{10} information—is a site called Nutrient Stew. Great information and links about CoQ_{10}, magnesium, selenium, vitamin C, fish oil, and prayer! If you're interested in CoQ_{10}, read this site as well.

I cannot say enough about Jon's site. I monitor it regularly and have promised Jon to do some topic reviews in the future.

Another heart failure site is run by my friend, Dr. Brian Jaski, called Heart Failure On-Line. It's a small site with some basics, and I'm sure it will grow over time. Reach it at

http://www.heartfailure.org

A site with more information but definitely a bit of commercial slant is Heart Information Network. Find it at

http://www.heartinfo.com

From here, you can go many places. Follow the heart failure links to find the Agency for Health Care Policy and Research guidelines, information on the Batista procedure, clinical trials, and an incomplete directory of clinics that offer outpatient infusions of inotropic agents.

If you are interested in finding some treatment algorithms, then I'd recommend the site from Boston University:

http://gopher1.bu.edu/COHIS/cardvasc/treatment/trtment.htm

Visit Medtronic to view a great site about dynamic cardiomyoplasty:

http://www.medtronic.com/cardiomyoplasty/bindex.html

And here's an update on the Batista procedure from the Cleveland Clinic:

http://www.ccf.org/news/971105.htm

Increasingly, many of the scientific sessions are available on-line for public perusal. In Canada, in 1996, there was initiated a superb program called the Cardiomyopathy and Heart Failure Summit. Virtually both the entire 1996 and 1997 congresses can be accessed on-line at

http://www.chfsummit.com

A good source of heart information, including the standard statistics, are at the Virtual Medical Center at

http://www.mediconsult.com/heart/

And finally, I must mention the web site for the Heart Failure Society of America at http://www.hfsa.org

We truly hope to be one of the best resources available on-line, so stay tuned.

SUPPORT GROUPS AND ORGANIZATIONS

If you want more information about pulmonary hypertension, then visit

http://www.phassociation.org

Find our more about depression at an AOL site. There must be other ways to get here, so keep trying

http://www.aol://4344:3147.pfizmain.21430283.532964492

If you want to check out your prescription drugs, there are many ways to do this, including

http://www.aol.com/netfind/timesavers/health.html#Prescription

OTHER COOL SITES

As you can tell by reading this book, I am a book aficionado. I don't think I'll ever enjoy pure electronic reading. I enjoy the touch and feel of books, so as long as they keep making them, I'll keep buying them. And the best place to buy I've found is Amazon. Check them out at

http://www.amazon.com

The *Merck Manual* is a great place to look up general health information. But an electronic, searchable one is even better. Lots of keystrokes here, but consider it exercise:

http://www.merck.com/!!u1wwqOh33u1wwqOh33/pubs/mmanual/html/
sectoc.htm

If you want to check out the latest clinical trials, then visit Center-Watch at

http://www.centerwatch.com

Access lots of the professional organizations' home pages and then take off from there. Among the best are:

http://www.chestnet.org/	American College of Chest Physicians
http://www.acc.org	American College of Cardiology
http://www.amhrt.org/	American Heart Association

These are chock-full of great information and are updated on a regular basis.

As I said, there is no way to put down all the sites I have read or ones that have some information worth reading. However, half the fun of using the Internet is doing the searches and seeing where they lead you.

As you can see, so much information is already available, with so much more coming, including interactive viewing, videoconferencing, and the like. Clearly, this is where we will get and share heart failure information in the future.

Hope to see you on the net!

Appendix I

Glossary of Heart Failure Terms

Angina pectoris Literally means pain in the chest, a symptom that often occurs when the heart muscle does not get enough blood. This is most often due to clogged coronary arteries, the arteries that carry blood to the heart muscle. Sometimes, however, a person can have poor blood supply to the heart and even suffer a heart attack without having angina pectoris.

Angiogram A test in which contrast material or dye is injected into an artery to see if the artery is narrowed or diseased. A coronary angiogram examines the arteries of the heart.

Angiotensin-converting enzyme inhibitor (ACEI) A drug that blocks a key enzyme reaction in the body so that another potent enzyme, angiotensin II, is not produced. Angiotensin II causes constriction or narrowing of the arteries, along with other detrimental changes.

Anticoagulation Inhibition of the coagulation or clotting process of the blood. Either weak hearts or hearts with certain irregular heartbeats, such as atrial fibrillation, are more likely to form blood clots, which can break off and spread to the lungs, brain, kidney, and so on. Medications such as aspirin or Coumadin are commonly used to "thin" the blood or prolong the clotting process, so that blood clots do not form in the heart.

Arrhythmia An irregularity of the heartbeat rhythm. Arrhythmia can originate in the upper chambers (atria) or the lower chambers (ventricles) of the heart.

Atrial fibrillation A heartbeat disorder whereby the two upper heart chambers fail to contract or squeeze in rhythm with the rest of the heart; thus, the heart loses the use of these two booster pumps.

Atrium (plural, atria) One of the two upper chambers of the heart, designated as the right atrium and the left atrium. The atria serve both as reservoirs of blood and as auxiliary pumping chambers. Blood from the body (arms, legs, and so on) returns to the right atrium; when the right atrium contracts or squeezes, it pumps the blood into the right ventricle, which is the main pump on the right side of the heart. From there, it is pumped up into the lungs, where oxygen is put into the blood. After the blood passes through the lungs, it goes to the left atrium, which then helps pump the blood into the left ventricle, or main pumping chamber on the left side of the heart, which sends the oxygen-containing blood back out to the body.

Beta-blocker A medication that blocks or inhibits the effect of body hormones on the tissues of the body. A beta-blocker can slow the heartbeat, among other things.

Blood pressure The pressure or force the blood makes in the arteries as it travels throughout the body. Blood pressure is a result of the contraction or squeeze of the heart plus the resistance maintained by the tiny muscles in all the arteries of the body. The systolic blood pressure (top number) is the maximal force generated with the squeeze of the heart. The diastolic blood pressure (bottom number) is the pressure that remains in the arteries as the heart relaxes or "reloads" for the next heartbeat.

Cardiac output A measurement of how much blood the heart pumps to the body per minute, usually expressed in liters per minute.

Cardiomyopathy A general term meaning there is something wrong with the heart muscle. When there is a specific cause, another term may be added, for example, ischemic cardiomyopathy, where the lack of blood (see ischemia) or a heart attack has caused the heart muscle problem. Another example is hypertensive cardiomyopathy, where the cause is hypertension, or high blood pressure.

Catheterization Passage of a catheter or tube into an artery or vein to make measurements. A cardiac catheterization records the pressures within the heart and lungs.

Congestive heart failure (CHF) See heart failure.

Coronary artery disease (CAD) CAD represents an entire spectrum of diseases due to blocked or clogged heart arteries, including angina pectoris, heart attack (myocardial infarction), or even heart failure due to poor blood supply to the heart muscle.

Cor pulmonale A special form of heart failure that involves only the right ventricle and is due to some problem or scarring in the lungs. Many patients with emphysema, or severe scarring and destruction of lung tissue due to cigarette smoking (one of the most common causes), can develop cor pulmonale, which also produces liver swelling, fluid in the abdomen, and leg swelling.

Cytokine Potent chemicals (usually proteins) produced by cells in the body that can affect heart muscle function. They may initiate an inflammation in the heart, stimulate the immune system, or both. Often, they have a negative or depressor action on heart muscle function.

Diastole The relaxing of the heart muscle as it "reloads" with more blood and prepares for the next heart contraction, or squeeze (see systole).

Digoxin A medication that can regulate the heart rhythm and help the heart muscle beat stronger.

Dilated cardiomyopathy A heart muscle problem in which the heart muscle becomes enlarged (dilated) and loses its elasticity (weakens).

Diuretic A medication that acts on the kidney to help rid the body of more salt and water, thus increasing urination.

Dyspnea The sensation that breathing is more difficult than normal.

Echocardiogram A noninvasive test that bounces sound waves off a heart to determine its size, structure, and function.

Edema Fluid, under excessive pressure, that leaks out of the blood vessels and gets into the tissue. Edema is commonly seen in the hands and legs, and also in the tissue of the lower back. Your doctor can also "hear" the fluid when it leaks into the lung tissue; this is called crackles or rales.

Ejection fraction The amount of blood the ventricles of the heart pump. The formula to calculate the ejection fraction is as follows: End diastolic volume (how much is in the chamber after it's fully filled or loaded) minus the end systolic volume (how much is left after the heart has emptied) divided by the end diastolic volume multiplied by 100 percent with each beat. For example, if the left ventricle holds 100 cubic centimeters of blood when it starts to pump, and if it holds 40 cubic centimeters at the end of the beat, it has ejected 60 cubic centimeters.

$$100 - 40 = 60$$
$$60/100 \times 100 = 60 \text{ percent}$$

This would be normal. In another example of an enlarged, weakened heart, where the end diastolic volume is 200 cubic centimeters and the end systolic volume is 150 cubic centimeters, then the ejection fraction would be

$$200 - 150 = 50$$
$$50/200 \times 100 = 25 \text{ percent}$$

Normal on the left side is about 50 to 60 percent, on the right side, 45 to 50 percent. When your doctor says your ejection fraction is 30 percent, then it is not one-third of normal but really one-half of normal.

Electrocardiogram   A simple test to check the electrical activity of the heart, including its rhythm, the presence of heart enlargement, or evidence of a prior or recent heart attack. An electrocardiogram is called an EKG or ECG.

Endomyocardial biopsy   A sampling of the heart muscle that can be looked at under the microscope. The heart tissue is obtained by passing a special instrument into a vein toward the heart. This is routinely done after a heart transplant to detect rejection of the heart.

Etiology   The cause of a certain condition. A heart failure etiology would be the medical condition that caused the heart to malfunction, such as a heart attack.

Familial cardiomyopathy   A rare form of heart failure that affects several members of a family. This is an inherited form of heart failure, usually of the systolic type.

Gallop   Abnormal sounds that the heart makes in a variety of conditions, including heart failure or hypertension. These sounds are so named because they resemble the rhythmic sound of a galloping horse's hooves as they strike the ground.

Heart   A chambered blood pump made out of muscle. Its job is to pump the blood around the body and supply oxygen or fuel and nutrients to the body tissues and organs.

Heart failure   A problem that can be induced by many different causes; it primarily means that the heart is not working as a pump as efficiently as it was meant to work.

Heart rate   The number of times or cycles the heart pumps per minute. Normal may vary from about fifty beats per minute to ninety beats per minute at rest.

Hypertension   An abnormal elevation of the blood pressure (see blood pressure).

Hypertrophic cardiomyopathy   A heart muscle problem in which there is excessive growth or too much heart muscle. Usually, the problem is with abnormal relaxation of the muscle (see diastole).

Idiopathic cardiomyopathy   A form of heart failure in which no specific cause can be determined.

Inotropic   Medical term meaning to improve the contraction or squeeze of the heart muscle.

Invasive   A test or procedure that involves entering the body, artery, or vein. For example, a cardiac catheterization involves placing tubes into the veins or arteries. An invasive procedure usually carries some risk, albeit small.

Ischemia   Medical term for lack of proper blood and oxygen supply to any tissue. A heart attack is ischemia to the heart muscle.

MUGA (or Radionuclide angiogram [RNA])   A nuclear medicine test that helps determine the ejection fraction or pumping ability of the heart.

Myocardial infarction   The medical term for a heart attack. The usual cause is a blocked coronary artery, which prevents blood and oxygen from nourishing the heart muscle.

Myocarditis   An inflammation of the heart muscle. This can be caused by viruses or bacteria, or may even result from an allergic reaction to medicines or drugs.

Myocardium   The medical name for the heart muscle.

Nocturia   Refers to getting up at night to urinate (see paroxysmal nocturnal dyspnea). Whenever the person with heart failure lies down, excess fluid may return to the heart; if the heart can sufficiently pump the blood down to the kidneys, urine is formed, which wakes up the person and signals him or her to go to the bathroom.

Noninvasive   Refers to a test or procedure that can be done without entering the body, such as an electrocardiogram or an echocardiogram. Usually involves minimal or no risk.

Norepinephrine   One of the body's stress hormones that is secreted in increased amounts in response to stress or danger, but returns to normal when the stress or danger has passed. With heart failure, the body senses a constant stressful state and the level of norepinephrine goes up and stays up. This elevation can be measured by a blood test and is one of the strong indicators of prognosis in heart failure patients.

Orthopnea   The sensation that breathing is difficult when you lie down.

Oxygen consumption (VO$_2$)   A measurement of how much oxygen the body is using. With exercise, for example, the body's need for oxygen increases, and hence the oxygen consumption measurement goes up. The status of the lungs, heart, blood, blood vessels, and muscle all affect this measurement. When a person has heart failure, the total amount of oxygen consumption is low, in part because the heart can't pump the blood and oxygen sufficiently. The peak or maximal oxygen consumption can serve as an indicator of the degree of heart failure.

Paroxysmal nocturnal dyspnea (PND)   Dyspnea is the sensation that breathing is more difficult, that one is short of breath. Paroxysmal nocturnal dyspnea, then, is the sensation of shortness of breath that comes on suddenly (paroxysm) at night (nocturnal). When people with heart failure accumulate extra fluid and are on their feet all day, the forces of gravity help push the extra fluid out into the tissues, thus forming edema (see edema). When the person finally lies down and the force of gravity is removed, the edema fluid eventually works its way back into the blood vessels and back to the heart. The weakened heart cannot sustain the extra fluid, and some backs up into the lungs, causing congestion. The fluid in the lungs prevents sufficient oxygen from getting in through the lungs, and shortness of breath results. Although this typically occurs at night, it can occur anytime—in the morning, for night workers, or even during a nap. Typically, PND occurs about thirty to sixty minutes after patients lie down. They may wake up coughing, gasping, or simply feeling uncomfortable. They may then sit on the edge of the bed, go to the bathroom, tuck an extra pillow under their head, or go to sleep on the sofa or in a recliner. With the head elevated, PND may not occur.

Prognosis A doctor's estimation, based on previous experience or medical studies, of what the outcome might be for an "average" patient with a particular disease. A prognosis may also involve an estimation of how long a person has to live.

Radionuclide angiogram (RNA) See MUGA.

Sinus rhythm The normal heart rhythm in which the upper heart chambers (atria) contract or squeeze in synchrony with the lower chambers (ventricles). Normally, the atria squeeze and help the blood pass to the ventricles; there is a wait for a fraction of a second while the ventricles fill completely, and then the ventricles squeeze. The exact coordination of the atria and ventricles is very important for maximal heart efficiency.

Swan-Ganz catheter A catheter, or tube, named after its two inventors, that is passed through the right-sided heart chambers and to the lungs to measure pressures within the heart and lungs.

Systole The contraction of the heart as it squeezes the blood out or the phase of contraction in the heart's two-phase cycle. The other phase, where the heart relaxes and "reloads" more blood and prepares for the next contraction, is called diastole.

Valve The heart valves help direct the flow of blood in a single continuous direction. There are four heart valves: the two that control the flow of blood between the atria and ventricles on the right and left are called the tricuspid and mitral valves, respectively. The two valves that direct the flow of blood away from the heart are called the pulmonic valve (which directs blood from the right ventricle into the pulmonary artery and into the lungs) and the aortic valve (which directs blood from the left ventricle into the aorta, which is the major artery of the body and leads to all the other arteries). These valves open and close with each heart cycle (more than 100,000 times each day!). They are quite durable but can be damaged by rheumatic fever, infection, and even aging. When the valve becomes too narrow and not enough blood gets through it, it is said to be stenotic. "Regurgitation" occurs when the valve leaks and blood flows back through the valve in the wrong direction.

Vasodilator A medication that dilates, or opens up, the arteries and veins of the body. This makes it easier for the heart to pump the blood, since the heart meets less resistance.

Ventricles The two main lower pumping chambers of the heart. The right ventricle has the job of pumping blood up to the lungs, where oxygen gets put into the blood. The left ventricle has the job of pumping blood to the whole body—the muscles of the arms and legs, the brain, the intestine, kidneys, and so on. Most heart failure results from some damage to the left ventricle, as would happen with a heart attack. However, the right ventricle alone can be weakened; most commonly, however, it is weakened when the left ventricle becomes weak and blood then backs up to the lungs and then to the right ventricle.

Appendix II

Resources for More
Information and Help
for Patients with Heart Failure

As I mentioned, the Internet is the new source for additional information. However, many people want to sit quietly and digest some of the important information about their heart and their condition. I would not have written this book originally if I thought there were sufficient sources of information for patients who suffer with heart failure and their families. I hope this book fills a gap, since that is its intended purpose. However, no book can be all inclusive, and I therefore want to list some of the other sources patients, families, and professionals can consult for more specific information, as well as for information on related topics.

The best place to turn to first is the Heart Failure Society of America (http://www.HFSA.org). This is now in my opinion the single best focused professional organization on heart failure. They also have a growing focus on patient education and most important, the information you will find there is bias free. To go directly to the patient information area, go to *http://www.abouthf.org*. Here you can sign up to get e-mail about new information and updates.

PROFESSIONAL ORGANIZATIONS

One place to turn to for more information is the American Heart Association. The national offices are in Dallas, Texas, but there are many local affiliates that can be found in most of the major cities within the United States. You should check your local phone book for the American Heart Association affiliate in your area, and a simple phone call will usually result in your receiving many free pamphlets full of information. The American Heart Association has a new, toll-free service, and simply by calling 1-800-AHA-USA1, you will be connected with the local office in your area. Otherwise, you can always write to the American Heart Association at 7272 Greenville Avenue, Dallas, Texas 75231. The American Heart Association publishes a variety of pamphlets; these are usually quite up-to-date and expertly done. Most of them concern general topics related to heart disease, for example:

1. *How to Make Your Heart Last a Lifetime.* This pamphlet describes general ways to take care of your cardiovascular health, including exercise, weight reduction, checking for diabetes, cutting the cholesterol out of your diet, lowering your blood pressure, and quitting smoking.
2. *A Guide to Losing Weight.* This pamphlet offers some good tips and a very good section on calorie counts.
3. *Save Food Dollars and Help Your Heart.* This is a good guide to good daily nutrition, with a focus on a low-fat diet.
4. *Sex and Heart Disease.* Although this pamphlet does not specifically address heart failure topics, it certainly is applicable to patients who have heart failure and is a good, quick read on this sensitive topic.

One of the books I have used for many years is one published by the American Heart Association of Metropolitan Chicago. This self-instructional booklet, *Congestive Heart Failure,* was written in 1985 and therefore is not absolutely up-to-date, but it has a very good introduction, some good diagrams of the heart, an explanation of what heart failure means, and excellent discussions of some of the common topics that need to be reviewed with heart failure patients. It also discusses a bit about medications and fluid and salt restriction. A similar booklet may be available from your local American Heart Association affiliate.

You may also call or write to the National Heart, Lung, and Blood Institute in Bethesda, Maryland, to inquire about specific research areas in a variety of cardiovascular diseases.

Other organizations that may have some general information on heart disease, aging, or both are the following:

American Geriatrics Society
770 Lexington Avenue
Suite 300
New York, New York 10021

American Association of Retired Persons (AARP)
601 E Street NW
Washington, D.C. 20049

Council of Geriatric Cardiology
777 West Putnam Avenue
Greenwich, Connecticut 06830

Again, these organizations may not have anything specific on the topic of heart failure, but they do have some other general good references. The American Association of Retired Persons, for example, has a variety of materials available, including an excellent folder entitled *A Path for Caregivers,* which is a good resource for families who end up providing a lot of care in the home.

Don't forget to use your local hospitals as a potential source for information. Each of the hospitals I work at has developed informative literature that is distributed to patients and their families to take home. You may also want to talk to the hospital social worker, who can provide additional information regarding the availability of home nursing services and visiting nurses, and who can frequently help arrange for Meals on Wheels, direct you to the local offices on aging, and serve as a liaison to some community-based services. For example, at one of our hospitals, social service workers frequently arrange free or low-cost transportation to and from subsequent office visits for all patients over the age of sixty-five who live within a certain community.

SUPPORT GROUPS

About ten years ago, I founded one of the first support groups for heart failure, I believe, within the entire country. The meetings specifically addressed the problems, questions, and concerns of the heart failure patient. Often, family members attended with the patient. We discussed many of the topics covered in this book, including fluid and salt restrictions, medication, and experimental trials. Unfortunately, that support group is no longer active, but others are springing up in various cities. Although I cannot guarantee what the content, leadership, or goals are for each of these support groups, if you find one in your area, I recommend checking it out to see if it is appropriate for you. Also, you might want to consider starting a support group yourself, perhaps with the help of the nursing or social service staff of your local hospital. I can tell you that the heart failure support group we ran combined an information session with a fifteen- to thirty-minute talk—on topics ranging from salt restriction to drugs to experimental therapies to communication skills—and a period of open communication. Almost all the patients felt relieved to know that others were in the same boat, and I think this is one of the major functions of any support group.

There are usually support groups affiliated with most heart transplant programs, but from my own experience, I would have to say that heart transplant support groups are generally not appropriate for most patients who have heart failure. However, it depends on the leadership of such support groups.

The Mended Hearts groups have multiple affiliates based at hospitals throughout the country. There are groups of people who provide encouragement and support at monthly meetings to all patients who have some form of heart disease. Most commonly, the members are patients who have suffered a heart attack or have gone through bypass surgery, but almost certainly, these groups include some patients with heart failure. In my experience, however, heart failure is not a topic commonly discussed at Mended Hearts meetings. You should check for the availability of such a group at your local hospital.

Because young people have other problems that aren't addressed in the Mended Hearts group, a wonderful organization called Young Hearts was founded several years ago by Julie Prochich. This organization, which started in Chicago, had multiple chapters throughout the United States. I'm saddened to say that because of loss of leadership, this organization no longer exists. In many ways it has been replaced by several CHF chat groups on the Internet. However, I do not think a chat group can ever replace personal interaction, and so I'm hopeful that this group might rebuild in the near future, since it addressed the special concerns of the younger patient that usually aren't available in other support groups I have seen.

DRUG INFORMATION

As I mentioned in Chapter 8, there are various sources for drug information, ranging from your local druggist to on-line computer services. I want to emphasize the importance of talking to your local pharmacist, using him or her as a resource. Also, libraries and bookstores offer a variety of books that discuss drugs and usage in general. The *Physicians' Desk Reference* is an excellent resource, albeit quite technical. This book is published by the Medical Economics Data Production Company in Montvale, New Jersey 07645-1742.

RECOMMENDED BOOKS

Many years ago, I was evaluating a heart transplant for a woman who had a rather severe form of heart failure. I had been called in by her primary cardiologist just shortly after he had told her, "I think you need a heart transplant—nothing else can be done for you." Although she was scared and somewhat taken aback by the notion that she might need a heart transplant, the woman kept her balance and sense of humor, and in the end, this fine, intelligent individual changed my perspective and approach to patients in general. She was one of the first patients who made me understand the emotions and thoughts involved in hearing the words *heart transplant* and *heart failure* for the first time. She wrote volumes of notes, which she shared with me, and I remember her words each day. I should tell you that she chose not to have a heart transplant, eventually entered one of our experimental drug protocols, and is doing exceedingly well today.

The main reason that I mention this patient at this time is because she was one of the first patients to ask me for something to read about heart failure. There were, of course, the pamphlets and books that we give to most patients regarding fluid and salt restriction, but she wanted more. She wanted to know some of the technical details regarding the results of the clinical trials, which drugs might be best for her condition, and how doctors really go about figuring out what a person's prognosis may be. I will never forget the day she came in for an office visit and ended up poring over my textbooks for about four hours. It was at that point that I realized that patients should read some of the medical textbooks, as long as they know up front that everything in the book does not apply to them, and as long as their doctor is available to interpret some of the information for them. Therefore, I am going to list here some medical textbooks that you may be able to find in your local library, a university medical library, or a hospital medical library. Perhaps your doctor will let you read his or her copy.

I wanted to recommend a couple of new books.

Aging Well. The Complete Guide to Physical and Emotional Health, written by Dr. Jeanne Wei and Dr. Sue Levkoff and published by John Wiley and Sons, 2000.

If you read any other book besides *Success with Heart Failure,* please read this one by my friend Dr. Jeanne Wei. She is one of the world's authorities on healthy aging and the book is filled with compassionate insight and scientific evidence as well as exceedingly practical information on managing medical bills, doctors visits, and so on. This book must be read by anyone who is aging or plans to age!

Another terrific book intended for doctors and nurses but readable by those of you who want to know some more of the basics of heart failure is *Basics of Heart Failure,* written by Dr. Brian Jaski and published Kluwer Academic Publishers in 2000. For most it may be a bit too much but I have many patients who could read it and understand a lot of it. Consider getting it as a holiday gift for your doctor or nurses (after you've bought them each a copy of *Success with Heart Failure,* of course!)

The Ciba Collection of Medical Illustrations, prepared by Frank H. Netter, M.D., edited by Frederick Yonkman, M.D., Ph.D., and published by Ciba-Geigy Corporation, West Caldwell, New Jersey, 1992. Most medical libraries have a copy of this collection, and volume 5 is the one regarding the heart. These are superb illustrations, and I believe most readers would find these fascinating.

A Color Atlas of Heart Disease: Pathological, Clinical and Investigatory Aspects, written by Drs. George C. Sutton and Kim M. Fox and published by Current Medical Literature, London. This is a fascinating book that describes pathological features of the heart in case histories of patients with a variety of cardiac diseases as revealed through such techniques as the electrocardiogram, the chest X ray, and the angiogram. I think this would be fascinating reading for most patients.

Congestive Heart Failure: Pathophysiology, Diagnosis, and Comprehensive Approach to Management, edited by Drs. Jeffrey Hosenpud and Barry Greenberg and published by Springer-Verlag, New York, 1994 (a new edition was be published in late 1998). This is one of the first medical textbooks dedicated to the topic of heart failure. This excellent resource is extremely detailed and current. It also has an exhaustive bibliography, so readers who are so inclined can find the original medical articles and go through them.

The Guide to Cardiology, edited by Dr. Robert A. Kloner and published by LeJacq Communications, New York, 1990. This is one of the more readable texts and has very good sections describing some of the common cardiac diseases and the tests that are done to diagnose them. This is available now in a soft cover and would be a good general heart book to flip through, as well as a good resource to consult for information on heart failure.

The Heart, edited by Dr. J. Willis Hurst and published by McGraw-Hill, New York, 1992. This is a standard general cardiology text with a good section on heart failure, one that would be quite comprehensible to most readers of this book.

Heart Disease: A Textbook of Cardiovascular Medicine, edited by Dr. Eugene Braunwald and published by W. B. Saunders, Philadelphia, 1994. This is a general cardiology textbook, but it has a superb section on heart failure. This book has recently been updated, and I would suspect that after reading

Success with Heart Failure, most people could easily read through the appropriate chapters in this textbook and understand most of the information presented.

The Living Heart Brand Name Shoppers' Guide, written by Drs. Michael De-Bakey and Antonio Gotto Jr., along with Dr. Lynn Scott and John Foreyt, and published by Master Media, Ltd., New York. There are a great many books on food and the heart, but I think this is the very best one. It has some general information about different food groups, but its strength is that it lists virtually every brand name of processed food, along with its calorie count, fat content, cholesterol content, and sodium content (so you need never exceed your two-gram sodium restriction again).

Love, Medicine and Miracles, written by Dr. Bernie S. Siegel and published by Harper and Row, New York, and *How to Live Between Office Visits,* also written by Dr. Bernie S. Siegel and published by HarperCollins, New York. I cannot overemphasize how important maintaining good mental health is for your success with heart failure. To my mind, no one has done more to raise the consciousness of patients and physicians alike and to teach them to communicate and explore their feelings together than Dr. Bernie S. Siegel. He has written several books—these two are my favorites—that primarily focus on his experiences in helping cancer patients deal with their emotions, but his messages of love and hope teach all patients, regardless of their medical condition, how to love life and regain health. His books can be read by virtually everyone, and I recommend them highly.

A Resource Directory for Older People, published by the National Institute on Aging. This book, which elderly patients with heart failure will find helpful, is the National Institutes of Health publication number 93-738. You can obtain more information on he book from the National Institute on Aging, Public Information Office, 9000 Rockville Pike, Building 31, Room 5C27, Bethesda, Maryland 20892. The phone number is (301) 496-1752. The publication service toll-free number for the National Institutes of Health is (800) 222-2225.

You Can Live with Heart Failure: What You Can Do to Live a Better, More Comfortable Life, written by Dr. Robert DiBianco for the Bristol-Myers Squibb Company. This booklet has been available for several years and is one of the best overall guides I have seen regarding heart failure. Dr. DiBianco, who practices in the Washington, D.C., area, is one of the country's outstanding cardiologists. The booklet, which contains some excellent points regarding heart failure, is distributed by the pharmaceutical company and may be available in your doctor's office.

MISCELLANEOUS

Because of the enormous interest and intensity of the problem with heart failure, several "Clinical Guidelines" have appeared for doctors. The very first set of guidelines published by the Agency for Health Care Policy and Research in 1994 is available widely on the Internet and directly through the federal government (publication no. 94-0612). They also published a well-written version of the guidelines for public consumption and should be a "must read" for all heart failure patients.

Another of the several sets of guidelines available that is also excellent is the one jointly published by the American College of Cardiology and the American Heart Association in 1995 and is again available via the Internet or directly through either organization. These guidelines are generalized distillations about diagnosis and treatment for only some of the patients with heart failure. Although I believe they provide good general recommendations, they cannot address anywhere near all of the pertinent questions for most patients with heart failure or address all the various situations different types of heart failure produce. Your doctors and nurses should be aware of these guidelines and know how they do or don't apply to your particular situation.

You should be aware that the American Heart Association holds a national meeting every November. Over 25,000 physicians, scientists, and nurses attend this meeting. Major advances in treating heart disease are frequently announced at this meeting and are then reported in the news media. The American College of Cardiology has its annual meeting in March each year, and this is another time when you are likely to hear about advances in heart failure care and treatment.

Finally, let me suggest the usefulness of signing up at your local hospital or community college to take an American Heart Association–sponsored cardiopulmonary resuscitation course (CPR) or one of the more advanced lifesaving courses. Not only will the skills you acquire help to allay the anxiety and sense of helplessness you may feel about the heart disease of a loved one, but you will feel a great deal of satisfaction in knowing that you possess knowledge and techniques that can be applied anywhere to save a life.

Finally, because of the increasing sophistication of medical consumers as well as rapid and open access via the Internet, I believe many patients want to read some of the original medical papers. You should certainly do this. I cannot list here all the papers that I think are useful, but I recommend a single current paper, "The Management of Chronic Heart Failure." I make all my young house officers read this well-written paper by Dr. Jay Cohn. It appeared in the *New England Journal of Medicine* in 1996, volume 335, pages 490–498.

Appendix III

Photographs of Hearts

In my office, I use several graphics to help explain to patients what heart failure is, what a heart attack is, where the left ventricle is, and so on. I suggest that you may well want to go to your library to get a general health book, medical book, or even *Gray's Anatomy* to review the basic structure of the heart.

I have included in this appendix several photographs of hearts demonstrating some form of heart failure. I hope that you see in these photographs the beauty of the heart as well as a clear image of the specific problem with each heart. I specifically want to thank Dr. William C. Roberts, who was the chief of the Pathology Branch of the National Heart, Lung, and Blood Institute, National Institutes of Health, Bethesda, Maryland, and who taught me so much about cardiac pathology and heart disease in general. It was in his laboratory that photographer Margaret Moore Bartlett captured on film the serious nature of heart disease.

The photographs on the following pages are accompanied by a brief description. You may want to consult the glossary as you study these photographs.

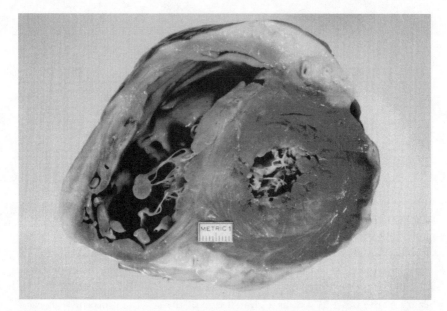

In this photograph we are looking up at a normal heart after a portion of the bottom two chambers has been sliced off. On the right side of the photograph is the left ventricle, with its thicker muscle, and on the left is the thinner right ventricle. Looking in the center of each ventricle, you can see portions of the heart valves, which direct the flow of blood in the heart. The one seen in the center of the left ventricle is the mitral valve, and the one in the right ventricle is the tricuspid valve. In all these photographs, the part of the heart at the top of the photograph is the part that faces the front of the body, and the bottom faces the back. As a point of reference, it is believed that when a person dies, almost without exception, the heart becomes fixed in the squeezing phase, or systole.

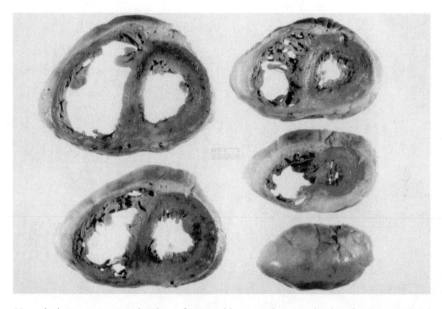

Here, the bottom pumping chambers of a normal heart, or the ventricles, have been removed and sliced into several layers. In each layer, the thicker left ventricle is on your right, and the right ventricle is on your left. You may notice a small amount of lighter fat on the surface of the heart, and this is normal. In this heart, there is no scarring, as from a heart attack; the chambers are not dilated or enlarged, and they are not excessively thickened.

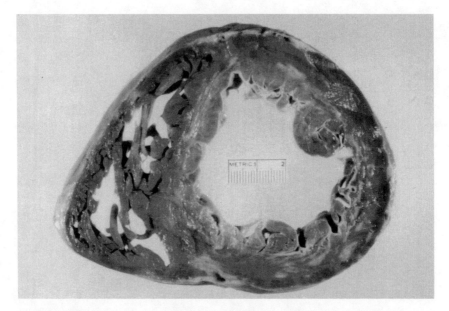

This photograph is a cross section of the ventricles, giving an example of systolic heart failure due to ischemic cardiomyopathy, or heart failure due to lack of proper blood flow to the heart through the nourishing arteries of the heart. This patient had at least two heart attacks. You can see several white flecks in the back portion of the left ventricle, which are areas of scar tissue from a heart attack. There are similar scars in the front portion of the left ventricle, which represents another heart attack. This patient had heart failure for many years, beginning just after the second heart attack. Compare the enlarged left ventricle with that of the normal heart. This is the kind of heart that cannot squeeze well; therefore, there is poor pumping of blood to the rest of the body.

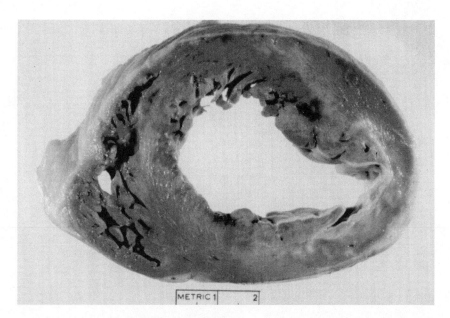

This is another example of an ischemic cardiomyopathy due to coronary artery disease. You see here a large area of white scar tissue on the far side of the left ventricle, which is called the lateral wall of the heart. The scar tissue represents a large heart attack that occurred in the past. Notice how thin this portion of the left ventricle is in comparison to the neighboring areas. Following a heart attack, the involved portion of the heart muscle becomes thinner, and this thinning occurs quite early. Therefore, in the first few days after a heart attack, that is, before strong scar tissue forms, the heart can indeed develop a hole or tear in it, and this is called a rupture of the myocardium. Fortunately, the scar that develops during the healing process is quite strong, and further ruptures do not occur. After a heart attack in which one portion of the ventricle is damaged, the adjacent areas take over the work; in fact, the muscle in these areas can thicken, or hypertrophy, which is why the area near the large scar in this photograph looks thicker than normal.

Now look carefully at the top portion of the left ventricle, and you will see a darker area of this muscle. This is a fairly recent heart attack. In fact, this patient had no symptoms of heart failure following the first heart attack, although it seems to have been a relatively large one. However, with the second heart attack, the patient came into the hospital severely short of breath and in congestive heart failure, and died shortly thereafter because of a serious irregularity of heartbeat.

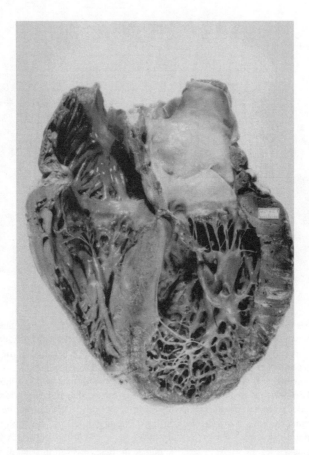

This is a view of the heart cut in half from top to bottom, with the front separated from the back. We are looking inside at the back portion and have a view of all four heart chambers. The atria are on the top, and ventricles are on the bottom. This patient suffered from dilated cardiomyopathy. There is no area of scar tissue or evidence of recent heart attack here, but notice that all four chambers are enlarged, which is typical in dilated cardiomyopathy. Although no cause for this patient's cardiomyopathy was ever found (and thus it is called idiopathic dilated cardiomyopathy), other cardiomyopathies, such as alcoholic or peripartum, could look identical to this. Note the delicate and beautiful valve structures.

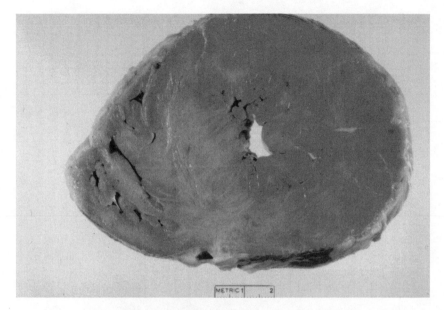

This is a transverse slice of the ventricles, demonstrating that heart failure is due to systemic hypertension, or high blood pressure. Notice how thick the left ventricle is. In response to the high blood pressure the heart faced with each beat, the muscle of the left ventricle thickened or hypertrophied in order to handle the load, much as the muscles of the arms or legs enlarge in response to a constant form of exercise.

Although you can't see them, there are also many small areas of scar tissue in this thick muscle. Compared to the normal heart, the actual cavity or space the blood would fill is much smaller. Because of the difficulty this kind of muscle has in relaxing, owing to its thickness, the small scars, and the relatively small chamber or cavity, it is harder for the blood to properly fill this chamber during the reloading period. As a result, not only does less blood get out to the body with each stroke or contraction but also there is a tendency for blood to back up into the left atrium. This situation is a good example of what is called diastolic heart failure. As is typical in this disease, this patient, who died at age sixty-eight, also had kidney malfunction and a stroke, all due to the high blood pressure.

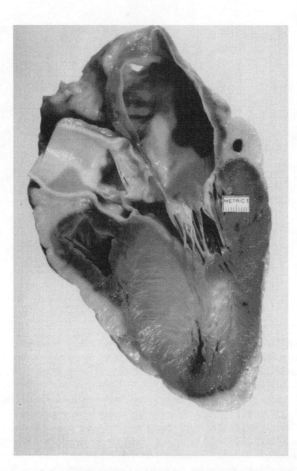

This is a photograph of a heart with a special form of diastolic heart failure known as hypertrophic cardiomyopathy. The heart has been sliced to show the left atrium and the left ventricle. The muscle of the left ventricle has grown excessively, especially the septum, or the portion that divides the right ventricle from the left. Notice how there really is only a very tiny cavity where the left ventricle normally is.

Patients can have multiple problems related to this disease, which can be hereditary, including heart failure with shortness of breath, both at rest and with exercise, chest pains, and serious irregular heartbeats. In fact, this patient was a twenty-three-year-old who died suddenly after climbing some stairs; other family members had the same disease.

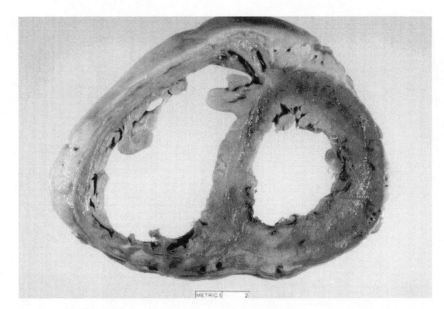

In this photograph, the left ventricle is actually quite normal in size and there is no evidence of a previous heart attack. Notice, however, that in this case, the right ventricle (on the left) is quite dilated. This person had what is called cor pulmonale. This is a form of heart failure in which the right ventricle becomes weak and dilated owing to some problem in the lungs.

The patient was a seventy-two-year-old with severe emphysema, or lung scarring due, in his particular case, to years of cigarette smoking. As a result of the lung damage, the pressure in the lungs rose, and each time the right ventricle pumped blood up to and through the lungs, it met a pressure that was more than 400 percent of normal. Eventually, the right ventricle failed to keep up this tremendous work, and right heart failure developed. The patient died with severe swelling of the liver, abdomen, and legs.

Appendix IV

Heart Failure and Exercise

The amount of materials I could add to this book is endless. At our Heart Failure Institute we created a simple but wonderful book that we give to all our heart failure patients. Much of this information you can get from our web site *(http://www.advocatehealth.com/sites/specialty/chf/patientdata.html)*. However, one thing patients always ask about is exercise and so we have created a new, simplified section on some of the basics of exercise. Obviously, there is so much more to be learned about exercise but these are some good starting places and so I have included these few pages and simple drawing for you to look at and enjoy!

Congestive Heart Failure & Exercise

Exercise is important for your treatment of CHF

Incorporating an exercise routine should be fun and part of the treatment plan for almost all CHF patients.

Exercise keeps your heart as strong as possible!!!!

Exercise Benefits

- Decreases fatigue
- Decreases shortness of breath
- Increases energy
- Increases endurance
- Decreases heart rate
- Improves quality of life

Guidelines For Exercise At Home

- Talk to your doctor about exercise.
- Suggested forms of aerobic of exercise to start are: walking, stationary bike-riding, or swimming.
- Always stretch before and after exercising.
- Wait at least one hour after meals before exercising.
- Medication should be taken as prescribed.
- Exercise at the time of day that you have the most energy – generally morning rather than afternoon.
- Begin slowly — 3 to 5 minutes, 3 to 5 time a week and gradually increase 5 – 15 minutes a week to reach a goal of 30 to 60 minutes per session, 4 to 6 time per week.

- Your walking speed will vary, depending on how you feel.
- Refer to the perceived exertion scale as a means of regulating your exercise.
- Avoid environmental extremes, such as: hot, humid, or cold. These extremes increase the demand on your heart.
- If your doctor approves, you may do some mild resistance exercises, starting out with 1 to 5 pound weights. (A low-sodium soup can is a good start.)

Stop Exercise If You Have

- Excessive shortness of breath
- Lightheadedness
- Sustained palpitations or irregular heartbeat that is not normal for you
- Chest pain
- Excessive fatigue during or after exercise

Things To Avoid

- Exercises causing chest pain, shortness of breath, dizziness, or lightheadedness
- Heavy lifting
- Extreme hot or cold
- Exercising when too hot or humid

Why Should You Stretch Before Exercising?

- Increase range or motion
- Warm up muscles for aerobic exercise
- Help prevent muscular injury
- Increase coordination
- Makes you feel better

Tips For Proper Stretching

- **DO NOT BOUNCE!**
- Hold stretch for at least 20 seconds
- Repeat each stretch 3 – 5 times
- You should not feel pain
- You should not feel fatigued

Perceived Exertion Scale

The following scale can be used to help determine when you have reached the level of exercise that will be most beneficial for you. You should stay in the range of the box.

1. Not tired at all

2.

3. A little tired

4.

5. Tired

6.

7. Really tired

8.

9.

10. So tired I can't go anymore

Sitting Warm-Ups

Shoulder Shrugs

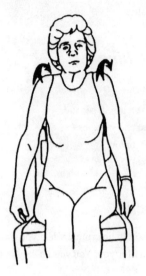

Arm Circles

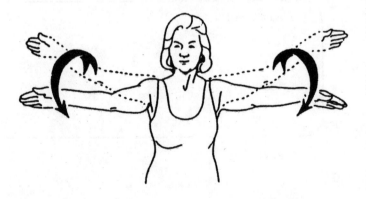

Knee Lifts

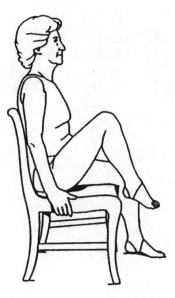

Ankle Curls

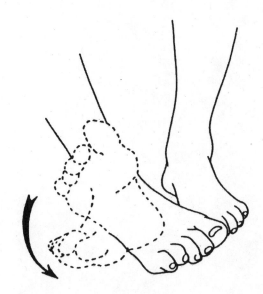

Sitting Warm-Ups (continued)

Ankle Bends

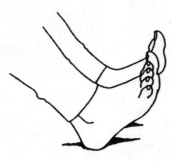 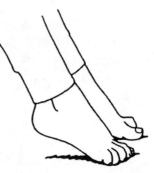

Standing Warm-Ups

Trunk Twists

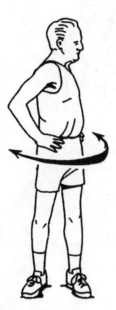

Toe Raises

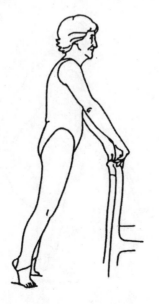

Stretches

Calf Stretch

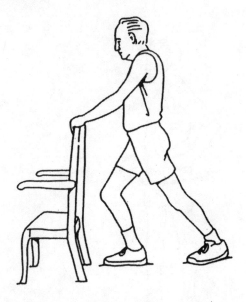

Quadriceps Stretch

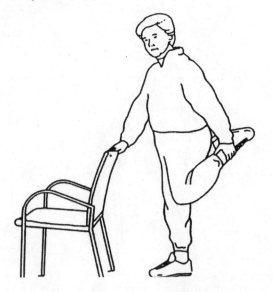

Activity Log

Share this log with your doctor and nurse.

Name: _____

Date	Total Time (Minutes)	Activity	How Do I Feel?

Date	Total Time (minutes)	Breed	How Do I Feel?

Appendix V

Feedback for Dr. Silver

The process of writing this book accomplishes one of my lifelong goals. As I said in the very beginning, my single motivation for writing this book has been the tremendous need my patients have expressed over the years. I started with the idea of simply putting together a brief pamphlet that patients could take home to share with their families and that would answer some of the common questions regarding heart failure. That pamphlet has blossomed into what I hope will be a useful but not burdensome book that will serve as a resource for patients, families, and health professionals.

On the other hand, I am 100 percent sure that I have not included every special situation or answered every single question that people may have about heart failure. And I am sure that my readers have had experiences in coping with their heart failure that many others could benefit from. I am not promising ever to write either an update or another edition of this book, but I would certainly welcome the opportunity to hear your comments about this book and to receive suggestions you may have from your own experiences dealing with heart failure. I promise at the very least to pass your ideas and suggestions on to my patients. I realized from the volume of mail I received after the first edition that I could not answer all the letters, let alone go through the medical records, medication lists, and so on that people sent.

Be assured that I read and appreciated every letter and note. You are all in my thoughts and I wish each of you well. Feel free to write to me, on the Internet, I hope. Otherwise, I'm sure our paths will cross somehow.

In the meantime, please feel free to write down whatever comments, thoughts, or suggestions you may have and send them directly to me at this address:

Marc Silver, M.D.
Success with Heart Failure
P.O. Box 2124
LaGrange, Illinois 60525

I wish you all success!

JNC VI Risk Stratification and Treatment Recommendations

- Determine blood pressure stage.
- Determine risk group by major risk factors and TOD/CCD.
- Determine treatment recommendations (by using the table below).
- Determine goal blood pressure.
- Refer to specific treatment recommendations.

Major Risk Factors
- Smoking
- Dyslipidemia
- Diabetes mellitus
- Age > 60 years
- Gender :
  - Men
  - Postmenopausal women
- Family history :
  - Women < age 65
  - Men < age 55

TOD/CCD (Target Organ Damage/ Clinical Cardiovascular Disease)

Heart diseases
- LVH
- Angina/prior MI
- Prior CABG
- Heart failure

Stroke or TIA
Nephropathy
Peripheral arterial disease
Hypertensive retinopathy

Blood pressure stages (mm Hg)	Risk Group A No major risk factors No TOD/CCD	Risk Group B At least one major risk factor, not including diabetes No TOD/CCD	Risk Group C TOD/CCD and/or diabetes, with or without other risk factors
High-normal (130-139/85-89)	Lifestyle modification	Lifestyle modification	Drug therapy for those with heart failure, renal insufficiency or diabetes Lifestyle modification
Stage 1 (140-159/90-99)	Lifestyle modification (up to 12 months)	Lifestyle modification (up to 6 months) For patients with multiple risk factors, clinicians should consider drugs as initial therapy plus lifestyle modifications.	Drug therapy Lifestyle modification
Stages 2 and 3 (≥160/≥100)	Drug therapy Lifestyle modification	Drug therapy Lifestyle modification	Drug therapy Lifestyle modification

Example: A patient with diabetes and a blood pressure of 142/94 mm Hg plus left ventricular hypertrophy should be classified as having stage 1 hypertension with target organ disease (left ventricular hypertrophy) and with another major risk factor (diabetes). This patient would be categorized as **Stage 1, Risk Group C**, and recommended for immediate initiation of pharmacologic treatment.

Goal Blood Pressure

<140/90 mm Hg	Uncomplicated hypertension, Risk Group A, Risk Group B, Risk Group C except for the following:
<130/85 mm Hg	Diabetes; renal failure; heart failure
<125/75 mm Hg	Renal failure with proteinuria > 1 gram/24 hours

SPECIFIC TREATMENT RECOMMENDATIONS

Lifestyle modification should be definitive therapy for some patients and adjunctive therapy for all patients recommended for pharmacologic therapy. Turn page over for a list of recommended lifestyle modifications.

INITIAL DRUG CHOICES

- Start with a low dose of a long-acting once-daily drug, and **titrate dose**
- Low-dose combinations may be appropriate

Uncomplicated Hypertension	Compelling Indications		Specific Indications for the Following Drugs:
Diuretics Beta-blockers	Diabetes type 1 (IDDM)	start with ACE inhibitor if proteinuria is present	(See Table 9 in JNC VI for specific indications) ACE inhibitors Angiotensin II receptor blockers Alpha-blockers Alpha-beta-blockers Beta-blockers Calcium antagonists Diuretics
	Heart failure	start with ACE inhibitor or diuretic	
	Myocardial infarction	beta-blocker (non-ISA) after MI; ACE inhibitor for LV dysfunction after MI	
	Isolated systolic hypertension (older patients)	diuretics (preferred) or calcium antagonists (long-acting DHP)	

From *The Sixth Report of the Joint National Committee on Prevention, Detection, Evaluation, and Treatment of High Blood Pressure.*
Arch Intern Med 1997; 157:2413-2446. NIH Publication No. 98-4080. For a copy of JNC VI, call the National Heart, Lung, and Blood Institute Information Center at 301-251-1222.

The JNC VI Guide To Prevention and Treatment of Hypertension Recommendations

Blood Pressure Measurement	Patient should: • Rest for 5 minutes before measurement. • Refrain from smoking or ingesting caffeine for 30 minutes prior to measurement. • Be seated with feet flat on floor, back and arm supported, arm at heart level. Clinician should: • Use the appropriate size cuff for the patient; the bladder should encircle at least 80 percent of the upper arm. • Use calibrated or mercury manometer. • Average two or more readings, separated by at least 2 minutes.
Primary Prevention	Encourage patients to make healthy lifestyle choices: • Quit smoking to reduce cardiovascular risk. • Lose weight, if needed. • Restrict sodium intake to no more than 100 mmol per day. • Limit alcohol intake to no more than 1-2 drinks per day. • Get at least 30-45 minutes of aerobic activity on most days. • Maintain adequate potassium intake—about 90 mmol per day. • Maintain adequate intakes of calcium and magnesium.
Goal	Set a clear goal of therapy based on patient's risk. Control blood pressure **to below:** • 140/90 mm Hg for patients with uncomplicated hypertension; set a lower goal for those with target organ damage or clinical cardiovascular disease. • 130/85 mm Hg for patients with diabetes. • 125/75 mm Hg for patients with renal insufficiency with proteinuria greater than 1 gram per 24 hours.
Treatment	Begin with lifestyle modifications (see primary prevention box) for all patients. Be supportive! • Add pharmacologic therapy if blood pressure remains uncontrolled. • Start with a diuretic or beta-blocker unless there are compelling indications to use other agents. Use low dose and titrate upward. Consider low dose combinations. • If no response, try a drug from another class or add a second agent from a different class (diuretic if not already used).
Adherence	• Encourage lifestyle modifications. Be supportive! • Educate patient and family about disease. Involve them in measurement and treatment. • Maintain communications with patient. • Discuss how to integrate treatment into daily activities. • Keep care inexpensive and simple. • Favor once-daily, long-acting formulations. • Use combination tablets, when needed. • Consider using generic formulas or larger tablets that can be divided. This may be less expensive. • Be willing to stop unsuccessful therapy and try a different approach. • Consider using nurse case management.

NATIONAL INSTITUTES OF HEALTH
NATIONAL HEART, LUNG, AND BLOOD INSTITUTE

Index

About the Author

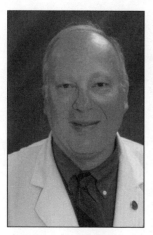

MARC A. SILVER, M.D.
Dr. Marc A. Silver is chairman of the Department of Internal Medicine, director of the Heart Failure Institute, and Associate Director of the Cardiovascular Disease Fellowship at Advocate Christ Medical Center in Oak Lawn, Illinois, and is a Clinical Professor of Medicine at the University of Illinois School of Medicine. He is one of the country's leaders in heart failure and has a long-established interest in heart failure, patient care, and nonpharmacologic therapy. His current research interests include the impact of heart failure education on functional status and quality of life, noninvasive hemodynamic monitoring, left ventricular assist devices as an alternative to heart transplant, and the newer inotropic and vasodilatory agents for decompensated heart failure, disease prevention, and resource utilization in cardiac disease. Dr. Silver has participated in over forty large-scale clinical trials as principal investigator and his scholarship and insights are reflected by his articles and abstracts published in *Journal of the American College of Cardiology, Congestive Heart Failure, New England Journal of Medicine, Transplantation,* and *Journal of Heart and Lung Transplantation.* He is coeditor-in-chief of *Congestive Heart Failure* and serves on the editorial boards of eleven professional journals including *American Journal of Cardiology, American Journal of Sports and Medicine,* and *Journal of the American College of Cardiology.* In addition, Dr. Silver is a reviewer for *American Heart Journal, American Journal of Cardiology, American Journal of Sports and Medicine,* and *Journal of Noninvasive Cardiology.* He is a fellow of the American College of Physicians, the American College of Cardiology, and the American College of Chest Physicians. His memberships include the American Federation for Clinical Research, the American Heart Association, and the American Medical Association, and he is a founding member of the Heart Failure Society of America. Dr. Silver received his MD degree from Rush Medical College in Chicago, Illinois, and he completed his residency at Rush-Presbyterian-St. Luke's Medical Center in Chicago, Illinois. He served as a medical staff fellow in the pathology branch of the National Heart, Lung, and Blood Institute, National Institutes of Health, in Bethesda, Maryland, and as a fellow in cardiovascular diseases at Rush-Presbyterian-St. Luke's Medical Center.